EAT TO BEAT DISEASE

HOW TO STARVE CANCER, WITHOUT STARVING YOURSELF.

BY:

Emy Skye

© **Copyright 2019 by Emy Skye All rights reserved.**

This document is geared towards providing exact and reliable information with regards to the topic and issue covered. The publication is sold with the idea that the publisher is not required to render accounting, officially permitted, or otherwise, qualified services. If advice is necessary, legal or professional, a practiced individual in the profession should be ordered.

From a Declaration of Principles which was accepted and approved equally by a Committee of the American Bar Association and a Committee of Publishers and Associations.

In no way is it legal to reproduce, duplicate, or transmit any part of this document in either electronic means or in printed format. Recording of this publication is strictly prohibited and any storage of this document is not allowed unless with written permission from the publisher. All rights reserved

The information provided herein is stated to be truthful and consistent, in that any liability, in terms of inattention or otherwise, by any usage or abuse of any policies, processes, or directions contained within is the solitary and utter responsibility of the recipient reader. Under no circumstances will any legal responsibility or blame be held against the publisher for any reparation, damages, or monetary loss due to the information herein, either directly or indirectly.

Respective authors own all copyrights not held by the

publisher.

The information herein is offered for informational purposes solely, and is universal as so. The presentation of the information is without contract or any type of guarantee assurance.

The trademarks that are used are without any consent, and the publication of the trademark is without permission or backing by the trademark owner. All trademarks and brands within this book are for clarifying purposes only and are the owned by the owners themselves, not affiliated with this document.

WHY YOU SHOULD READ THIS BOOK

Though we have all heard the term "Cancer" through many sources, the exact facts and details of the disease is not very widely known. Cancer is one of the world's deadliest diseases and is a completely curable if detected at an early age. It is therefore a must to possess awareness about it and this book is a consolidation of the facts and details related to this disease.

Cancer patients as a group typically have to suffer through months if not years of ongoing treatment. In far too many cases, after subjecting themselves to very unpleasant treatment protocols, they end up having to resign themselves to the fact that it didn't work.

That is a very depressing reality and a dire predicament that a large number of cancer victims have to resign themselves to coping with. All that pain and suffering and still not cancer free.

What can they or should they do at that point when all seems lost? In most cases it comes back to how accepting they have become to their likely fate. Many spend their last months preparing for the inevitable by saying goodbye to loved ones. Many others attempt to complete their version of a "wish list." By trying to do as many things that they have long wanted to do but just couldn't find the time or motivation to get done.

Others go into a deep depression, withdraw into a shell and never quite come to terms with their fate. Yet, others choose to be very active participants in their outcome and are committed to try to somehow fight a war to the bitter end with their cancer.

This last group who seem to fervently believe in hope and self determination tend to be very aggressive at researching and trying to find information that will give them a real chance at beating their cancer. They know of and believe the existing stories of cancer victims who were determined to fight cancer to the bitter end and won!

Luckily enough for that group, over the last seventy years a treasure trove of good research has been done on cancer. Coming out of that research and clinical trials are some really good data that gives real hope. Unfortunately, the problem is, getting effective treatment protocols from the research lab into clinical trials and ultimately to frontline physicians takes a very long time. In some instances a decade or longer. Most cancer victims don't have the luxury of waiting years for these new treatments to make it to the frontlines in the war against cancer. They are now measuring time in terms of months not years!

This book explores what a cancer victim can do to take advantage of the seventy years of clinical research that has occurred. With the objective being to use that knowledge in their fight against the disease.

TABLE OF CONTENTS

Introduction 1

Chapter 1: Your Muscle Mass - Critical To Cancer Prevention & Recovery 15

Chapter 2: How To Starve Cancer Without Starving Yourself 17

Chapter 3: Common Types Of Cancer................................ 33

Chapter 4: How To Prevent Cancer..................................... 47

Chapter 5: Understanding Colon And Rectal Cancer 59

Chapter 6: Beat Cancer & Power Up Your Immune System 64

Chapter 7: Antioxidants, Acids, Alkali And Cancer............... 70

Chapter 8: Membrane Sensors And Transporters 77

Chapter 9: In Early Cancer... 81

Chapter 10: Beating Cancer With Natural Food That Supports Life.. 88

Chapter 11: Fda Consumer Journal's Top 20 Fruits, Vegetables, And Fish... 104

Chapter 12: Fundamental Features Of Oral Hygiene......... 115

Chapter 13: Common Oral Hygiene Pitfalls: How To Overcome Them.. 119

Chapter 14: The Perfect Diet Plan: Eat Lean Protein Meals And Forget The Unbalanced Diet...................................... 122

Chapter 15: Low-Fat, High-Protein Meals - 7 Tips For A Healthier Body 126

Chapter 16: How Is The Quality Of Mid-Day Meals Maintained..129

Chapter 17: Balance Your Life - Having A Balanced Diet....132

Conclusion..134

INTRODUCTION

The cure for cancer is still some way off but it is something that science expects to happen possibly within the next few decades; medical research continues to advance in it's war with this disease that plagues humanity. The cure will come eventually and the world will rejoice that this awful disease that can strike anyone at any time has been silenced. The reasons cancer is triggered in the body are only theories as it can be caused by many things.

First off it is a good idea to understand exactly what cancer is and try to ascertain whether it is hereditary or something you can acquire. Firstly, it is a disease that starts as a group of abnormal cells that continue to divide; they cross over to other cells and sites of the body continuing to grow and divide.

The malignant property of cancer differentiates it from benign tumors which limit their growth and do not invade or metastasize. Some benign tumors, however, are capable of becoming malignant. It causes more deaths per population than any other illness and the older you get the more prone you are to contracting the disease; Statistics show that the number of people cancer kills globally each year is about 13 in every one hundred. Cancerous cells may have been transformed by radiation or poison for example and this creates genetic abnormality in those cells which then continue to grow and divide.

Although genetic abnormalities may be caused by it they may also be randomly acquired through problems in the body's DNA replication; a genetic trait may be inherited and thus present in all cells from birth. It would seem some people are more susceptible to it than others and it may be their genetic makeup and their exposure to certain carcinogens that is responsible.

Owing to this ongoing, worldwide research, we do actually know a considerable amount about cancer even if we are some way from finding a complete and consistent cure. More information is being gathered about all illnesses and why some people are more prone to certain conditions. Knowledge like this could enable more people avoid contracting cancer in the first place.

The food you eat on a regular basis will have an effect on your health, especially in the future. Some believe it may even be causing a large number of cases in certain groups of people. People are generally eating too much of the wrong things such as an excess salt intake, too much saturated fat and certain dairy produce. Studies have shown that there is a connection between dairy produced calcium and prostrate cancer.

Cancer is not gender specific, it does not have preferences as it will invade just about every part of the human body and organs. No one is safe. Sometimes the disease is only picked up through routine screening. Usually the cancer is at an early stage and a person may have a better chance of being cured. the number of different types of cancer that can be treated has increased dramatically in recent years with so much intensive research being carried out. Advancements in medical techniques mean that cancer in many cases can be treated and often completely cured; it is only a matter of time before a complete cure is discovered.

The states of mind influence the body, the immune system, and perhaps the course of disease.

In many aspects of our lives the response to the problem is much more important than the problem itself. Hopelessness and helplessness keep us from moving forward into action and healing. Maybe it is how we interpret stress, as either an oppressor or motivator that is the key. Once diagnosed with disease stress is a factor we can control. Perhaps inspiration lies beyond our current beliefs, our paradigms, and our bonds, in a world of miracles, wonder, and unlimited possibilities.

On the deepest level we have tenacity for survival. When we are immobilized by fear of pain, loss, dependency, disfigurement or non-existence our lifeline is action. Action taken daily towards healthy eating, proper exercise, setting strong boundaries, clearing up the muddle, connecting with our spirituality, and exploring who we truly are, can renew our sense of hope.

The physician and his team are your trusted gatekeepers. No form of disease is hopeless. All forms inspire new research and solutions. Be the hero in your own life reborn to all your potentialities.

Get engaged in every aspect of your life, body, mind, and spirit, to achieve optimal health. Involve a partner, or teams of partners. Teams beat disease.

Is your soul or spirit self a friendly play to be? Are you in sync with your connectedness to the world? Have you questioned and explored your own sacred excellence? Spirituality is a way of looking at yourself and others that surrenders you to a greater power. A healthy sense of spirituality keeps you in flow emotionally and may transcend to your physical body.

Your body is the expression of your inner self. Worship and honor it through exercise and wholesome eating. With just three to five hours of physical activity a week at a moderate pace women with breast cancer decreased their risk of relapse.* Get those endorphins, your natural opioids working for you.

Customize your exercise program based on the diagnosis, the treatment, your energy level, and the recommendations of your physician. Once your physician has cleared you to exercise consider the five components of fitness in the plan.

Your mind projects the energy within you. When you have clarity of what you want, what you value, and what you worship, you can live a joy filled life by integrating these components.

Come to a simpler life, invest in yourself and discover your unique values. Fulfillment comes from being your true self, maintaining and reflecting that self, and loving it. Discovery takes action and action grows hope.

There is a lot of myth and misconceptions surrounding healthy eating amongst people that requires solving. Healthy eating is not about maintaining strict and unrealistic diet plans and nutritional philosophies, keeping your body weight to a minimum or depriving yourself of the foods that you love. It is rather about staying happy and light and keeping yourself as healthy as possible by eating smart, learning to modulate your diet and knowing what works for you and then using it to your benefit. Your food choices aren't just about what you eat but how you eat it and help to defend your body against diseases like heart diseases, diabetes and cancer. A complete and wholesome nutrition not only enhances your fitness but also boosts your energy, sharpens your memory and improves your mood. Therefore reinvent your diet and learn how to create and maintain a healthy lifestyle sans diseases in a few simple ways:

Modifying your diet plan and expecting results overnight is unrealistic. You must realize that creating a good lifestyle requires time and patience, so start from scratch and move step by step and instead of being busy counting calories after every meal that you take learn to include all the essential food groups such as carbohydrates, vegetables and fruits, proteins and dairy products in your meals. Too much or too little of nothing is good and the key to a healthy diet lies in moderation and so do not overeat. Enjoy the food that you're eating because this will improve your metabolism and thus your body's ability to burn calories.

Maintaining a proper body weight is essential for healthy living. Your right weight depends on a variety of factors such as sex, height, age and heredity. Excess body fat can cause heart diseases and diabetes etc; similarly very low weight can cause fatigue, depressions and other diseases. Hence activities to facilitate weight loss should be followed for people with excess body weight.

Exercise is a dieter's best friend. It not only burns those extra calories but also improves your body's metabolism thus not only helping you to beat the bulge but also reduces the risk of various diseases. Research shows that three 10-minute spurts of exercise per day is equivalent to one 30 minute workout so start by taking the stairs instead of the elevator and going for long walks.

Do not deprive your body of its share of rest and reduce stress and stress related activities in your life. Enjoy every moment and lead a happy life without worries. Remember that you can never lead a healthy lifestyle if you're mental and psychological condition is unhealthy and if you have space for worries and depressions in your life. Thus in a nutshell the path to fitness and healthy leaving is simple if you know what to do and how to do it. Control your diet, gain optimum nutrition and exercise regularly to achieve weight loss and lead a happy and healthy life.

The idea that eating natural foods can contribute to preventing and healing cancer is often pushed to the back burner. However this could be a winning solution. In fact, in the face of runaway cancer statistics this should be one of your first considerations. Of course to do this you will have to adopt a fresh food is best attitude.

Consider your attitude. Attitude is determined by your mind set and we have been condition by our philosophy of capitalism and the constant commercial chatter to first seek help from something that will increase profits. Cancer treatment is becoming the fireworks of big profits in this arena.

You owe it to your health and well being to consider these three choices that will support you in your quest to greatly increase your chance to beat cancer and win.

These foods all boost and bring stamina to your disease fighting system, your immune system.

Grapefruit, lemons, limes oranges and kiwi all contain high levels of Vitamin C which will jump start your immune system. Vitamin C loses its healing properties when manipulated in the process of extraction and being processed for packaging to help prevention of cancer, so fresh is best. Your new attitude or mindset will be to not use any canned or bottled goods that contain Vitamin C.

Sure it is convenient and profitable to get gallons of citrus juice. Or pick up canned beverages with large amounts of vitamin C. However I know from having to work with this vitamin in a scientific lab how quickly it loses its potency.

Fresh citrus eaten or juiced and consumed immediately is best for your quest to support your immune system. Kiwi is very high in Vitamin C and can be added to fresh salads. Although fruits with Vitamin C taste acid it actually keeps body fluids alkaline and this can keep the hydrogen Ion concentration of your blood into the range that is not favorable to the support of cancer cells. With these errant cells under control your healthy cells will thrive and there will be a boost in production of your killer immune cells. So to get major benefit from this fighter, citrus must be eaten very fresh with no added ingredients such as sweeteners like sugar or its enticing substitutes. You don't have to read the label when eating fresh fruit or freshly squeezed juice. Easy!

Next seek out food with minerals that enhance immune function and also keep fluid in body organs balanced. Here again is where your fresh food attitude counts... minerals that support immune function are vitamin E, selenium, copper and zinc. Again getting these minerals and vitamins from your fresh food diet is more effective than supplementation. There is a basic synergy in fresh vegetables that the body can use to quickly get benefit from small portions, which is not available in pill form.

Gather fresh vegetables that are high in vitamin A and loaded with minerals and make a broth to drink throughout the day. Make this drink to replace coffee, sodas, and highly sweetened juice drinks even if it is the latest designer drink that a celebrity is using.

Most commercial drinks are highly acid forming and cancer thrives in this acidic condition. Choosing green leafy vegetables, such as kale and mustard greens, cabbage and roots like carrots, onions and ginger and turmeric will add trace minerals that will support your blood and brain chemistry, increase body alkalinity and upgrade your immunity.

With these choices, your improved immunity will do a superb job and win the fight for you. This action along with your new mind set can also boost your assurance of successful recovery.

The third thing you can do is to enhance your chances for complete recovery by upgrading your oxygen capacity. Gather foods that contain large amounts of chlorophyll, like spirulina, wheat grass and seaweed. Low oxygen levels in cells can promote the growth of cancer cells. Along with acidic blood most cancer patients have low levels of oxygen. Spirulina can be easily found in dried powder form in the bulk spice section of health food grocery stores. It is worth seeking out simply because it will help regulate the tumor destroying activity of your immune system's natural killer cells. Spirulina can be added to a well crafted smoothie or blended into fresh juice. And you have been led to believe that you have to fight cancer... Another benefit of theses green foods is that they will also help to clear toxic byproducts from cells.

Eating seaweed is an ancient practice of Japanese and Chinese cultures. Dried seaweed is soaked in a small amount of water. After it absorbs the water it is ready for dressing and eating. Usually this salad is eaten with other immune enhancing foods like ginger and mustard. Notice that this is quick easy and requires no cooking. Try eating this in an Asian restaurant. I discovered this wonder food with one of my Japanese friends in Hawaii and have been enjoying its benefits ever since.

Other green foods that can be eaten fresh are alfalfa, wheat grass and broccoli sprouts. The dressing for these should be very simple and fresh. An appropriate dressing would have fresh lemon or lime juice, and grape seed, sesame or walnut oil and no sugar added.

Vitamin C found in lemon and limes have healing properties when fresh and not manipulated in the process of extraction and being processed for packaging, so fresh is best.

The promise of this fresh is best attitude brings so much for so little effort it is almost hard to believe. But go ahead, give it a try and watch your health and your peace of mind soar. As your stress level plummets. You will also be ahead of the game in beating cancer and winning the fight.

What is Integrative oncology? The science of combining both medical, conventional treatments of cancer mixed with biobehavioral techniques, nutrition, supplementation, exercise, limiting or eliminating the many poorer lifestyle habits such as being sedentary, a poor diet that is supportive of cancer growth, alcohol & smoking.

Living cancer free - goes a long way to slow down aging, prevent diabetes, prevent heart disease... and feel extremely energetic, focused & productive.

People don't die from Cancer - they die from complications & consequences of the disease. An inflammatory cascade, biochemical toxicity, pneumonia, embolism... Therefore optimizing the biochemical environment & helping people thrive through the treatment with integrative oncology (those lifestyle habits nutrition, & exercise) is just as important as zapping tumors.

Omega 6s make you sick. Omega 3s & 9s make you healthy. Stick to walnut, olive, avocado, canola, rice bran

& sesame oils. Watch the smoke point, no reusing oil.

Dietary choices have a massive impact on the body's biochemistry - creating either an environment of cancer hospitality or hostility

5kg of weight gain in a breast cancer patient increases mortality by 14%

Alcohol: anything more than a tiny amount of alcohol can fuel cancer and increase recurrence, progression & mortality. Breast cancer - any alcohol is the enemy. BTW - very small amount = 1 glass per week. Alcohol is putting lighter fluid on a fire. Again - all of us have cancer - alcohol encourages replication of cancer cells. Alcohol takes advantage of sparks we all have- we all have periodic immune suppressions - don't add lighter fluid.

A diet of less than 20% fat, has a 24% reduction in the risk of reccurrence - that is on par with tamoxifen - or any drugs available for treatment of breast cancer & other tumors. Unfortunately, most oncologists do not even discuss diet details - its just "eat a healthy diet".

Consuming the right fats, can reduce the recurrence & mortality from many cancers - the EPA/DHA ratio - eat your cold water fish! 25g of flax seed a day - another great choice for getting your fatty acids.

Cancer cells love sugar! One of the thousands of reasons to ditch sugar, refined flours, aka empty carbs. These cancer promoters raise insulin - fuel that cancer!

Get an assessment & profile to know the right foods to create an anticancer environment suited to you. But lots of berries, eat a rainbow, vegetables, plant based proteins, beans & lentils...

EXERCISE! Keep active through out the day. Walking 6 hours a week can drop colon cancer mortality by 60% - one of many examples - I don't care how busy you are at your computer - there is no excuse. You don't have to go to a gym. Aerobic exercise for 10 minutes before chemotherapy - can cut the toxicity by 50% - Wow! But yes, speak to a cancer trained exercise professional for the right type of exercise

Biobehavioral aspects of cancer - psychological reduction of stress for immunity - Breast cancer recurrence rates reduced by 45%, mortality 56%, mortality all causes by 49%. Don't ever underestimate the power of the mind.

You smoke? Stop! Success rates of smoking cessation are far greater with a counsellor rather than the dance of quit relapse.

Excess adiposity - body fat - again - much better success rates when done as part of a take control health modification program with trained health coaches. Proper guidance with a health coach can help you ditch the yo yo. Retraining our minds, our attitude, self empowerment are equally as important as the diet and exercise

Transforming our biology: our ecosystem - do we

support a malignancy, or do we inhibit cancer growth? Comprehensive blood & tissue testing necessary to measure individual markers of cancer resilience.

This is why Integrative Oncology is a must in cancer treatment. Mapping patients - obtaining markers from cancer patients to help focus in on individualized cancer treatments. There are NO TWO PATIENTS WITH THE IDENTICAL DISEASE. Treatments of the disease are very dependent on the biochemical markers & tissue testing, genomic related biomarkers - very different story from one patient to another. Playing piano chords on patients let's play a symphony not a cacophony.

Assessments in biobehavioral aspects: psychological & emotional profiling. False hope over false hopelessness - the latter creates the biology that supports the disease.

CHAPTER 1
YOUR MUSCLE MASS - CRITICAL TO CANCER PREVENTION & RECOVERY

Circadian health - so much more than getting enough sleep. Known as a critical factor in health biology to kill cancer.

An anti inflammatory environment - basics of cancer prevention. Inflammatory biochemistry is a tumor promoting toxic soup. Again, diet & exercise - huge here. A cancer prevention diet, not a fad diet, a very specific cancer prevention diet that protects us from all chronic diseases.

Vitamin D - Unfortunately our RDIs have not targeted this number for cancer prevention. Look into Vitamin D as part of a complete lifestyle modification program & transforming our biology.

Chronomodulated chemotherapy - Both cancer cells & cancer drugs are time dependent - Each drug has a personality of its own and better given at certain times of day, at different rates. This technique provides up to an 87% reduction in toxicity of the drugs - very often the drug is the limiting factor in treatment because of drug tolerance. Making it through a treatment is paramount to cancer recovery.

Summarizing tips: Eat a plant based diet as much as possible, smaller cold water fish, a variety of exercise, sleep in a blacked out room (don't suppress those melatonin levels!), don't fall asleep to TV, stress management, meditation or prayer twice per day to calm & focus. "You can't build a strong foundation on top of quicksand"

CHAPTER 2
HOW TO STARVE CANCER WITHOUT STARVING YOURSELF

What is Cancer?

The term 'Cancer' refers to any one of a large number of diseases in which a group of cells show an abnormal development with an uncontrollable division beyond the normal limits. They have the ability to intrude and destroy adjacent body tissues. Cancer cells have the ability to spread throughout the body via lymph and blood, thus destroying the healthy tissues (process known as invasion).

All the cancers begin in the basic unit of life - the cell. Normal cells in a body have the ability to grow and divide in a controlled way to produce more cells as per needed to keep the body healthy. When the cells become old or damaged, they die and get replaced with new cells. If and when this normal process gets disturbed then cancer gets initiated. In a normal process, old cells die after a certain period of time and are replaced by new cells. But in a cancerous state, new cells keep on developing while old cells do not die when they should thus leading to a mass of tissue known as a tumor

Cancer is not a single disease but a class of diseases which are typically characterized by random and out-of-control growth in the human body cells. These random cell growth leads to invasion of other normal cells around them leading to their destruction. The cancerous cells divide in an uncontrollable fashion and form lumps or tissue masses known as tumors. These tumors affect the body part where they grow and disrupt their normal functioning. The cancerous cells also spread to other parts of the body through blood or lymph and cause further cell destruction.

Oncologists are physicians or researchers who study about the diagnosis, treatment and sure of cancer. The study of cancer is by itself known as oncology.

Cancer is An abnormal growth of cells which tend to proliferate in an uncontrolled way and, in some cases, to metastasize (spread).

Cancer is not one disease. It is a group of more than 100 different and distinctive diseases.

Cancer can involve any tissue of the body and have many different forms in each body area. Most cancers are named for the type of cell or organ in which they start. If a cancer spreads (metastasizes), the new tumor bears the same name as the original (primary) tumor.

The frequency of a particular cancer may depend on

gender. While skin cancer is the most common type of malignancy for both men and women, the second most common type in men is prostate cancer and in women, breast cancer.

Cancer frequency does not equate to cancer mortality. Skin cancers are often curable. Lung cancer is the leading cause of death from cancer for both men and women in the world today.

Benign tumors are NOT cancer; malignant tumors are cancer. Cancer is NOT contagious.

Cancer is the Latin word for crab. The ancients used the word to mean a malignancy, doubtless because of the crab-like tenacity a malignant tumor sometimes seems to show in grasping the tissues it invades. Cancer may also be called malignancy, a malignant tumor, or a neoplasm (literally, a new growth).

Cancer is not a new dub for the people breathing in the 21st century. It is as recurrent as our day to day usual activities. Every year about a million of new cases of cancer are diagnosed throughout the world. Most people loose their lives because of cancer. Treatment are available but there is still no 100% surety of recovery from cancer. Cancer influences almost every organ of human body transfiguring it into ruins in later stages.

Truly speaking cancer is not a single disease, but a heterogeneous group of disorders that are characterized by the presence of cells that loose control on normal cell division. Cancer cells divide rapidly and continuously resulting in formation of tumours that eventually strike healthy tissues. These tumourous cells travel across healthy cells creating tumours in them. The most frequent cancers include cancers of breast, lung, prostrate, blood, colon, rectum, pancreas, liver etc.

Formation of Tumour

Basically normal cells grow, divide, mature and die in response to a complex set of internal and external signals. A normal cell receives both stimulatory as well as inhibitory signals which are responsible for its growth, division and maturation. In case of a cancer cell, these signals get disrupted, so the cell divides abnormally at a higher rate. After losing normal control, the cancer cell loose its normal shape and forms a distinct mass what we call a 'tumour'. If the cells of a tumour remain localized it is termed a 'benign tumour' but if the cells invade other tissues, the tumour is termed as 'malignant tumour'. Cells that travel to other sites of the body, they form secondary tumours and have undergone 'metastasis'.

Cancer- The Genetic Aspect

Cancer is the culmination of abnormal cell growth so needs attention both publicly as well as scientifically. A number of theories have been put forward regarding cancer but now researchers realize that most if not all cancers arise from the defects in DNA> Previous views recommend the genetic origin of cancer. Many agents like ionizing radiations, chemicals that we come across result in episode of mutations that cause cancer. Some cancers are often syndicated with chromosomal abnormalities, about 90% of people with chronic myeloid leukemia bear a reciprocal trans location between chromosome 22 and chromosome 9> These observations accord clues for the genetic origin of cancer. In 1971 Alfred Knudson proposed a model for defining the genetic basis of cancer. His model id designated as 'Knudson multistep model of cancer', he was studying retinoblastoma- a cancer that develops in only one eye but occasionally appears in both> Knudson's proposal highlights that cancer is a multistep process requiring several mutations, if one or more mutations are inherited additional mutations are also obligatory to disclose a cancer and the cancer will run in families. His model has been confirmed today.

Cancer starts when a single cell is encountered with mutation and results in its abnormal growth. This cell divides and forms a clone of cells each carrying same mutation. An additional mutation that occurs in any of the clone cells may further enhance adroitness of these cells to burgeon and cells with both mutations become dominant. In this process, depicted as clonal evolution, the tumour cells gain more mutations that allow them to become increasingly aggressive in their proliferate aspects. The rate of clonal evolution depends upon the frequency of occurrence of new mutations. The genes that regulate DNA repair have also been found to get mutated in progressive cancer stages and inherited disorders of DNA repair are usually depicted by intensified incidences of cancer. Normally DNA repair mechanisms eliminate many of the mutations but cells with defective DNA repair systems are more likely to remain mutated including the genes that regulate cell division. Many cells are aneuploid and hence accelerate cancer progression.

Are Environmental Factors Also Responsible For Cancer?

Smoking is a good paradigm of environmental factor confronted with cancer strongly. Other environmental factors incorporate certain types of chemicals such as benzene (industrial solvent), benzo [a] pyrene (cigarette smoke), polychlorinated biphenyls (transformers and capacitors). Ultraviolet light, ionizing radiations, viruses are other carcinogens associated with cancer. Most environmental factors cause somatic mutations that quicken cell division.

Genes Contributing Cancer

The signals that regulate cell division fall under two categories: molecules that speed up cell division and others that inhibit it. Because cell division is perturbed by these two factors, cancer can arise from mutations in any of these two factors. Mutations in stimulatory genes are usually dominant and are termed 'oncogenes'. Oncogenes were first identified cancer causing genes discovered by Peyton Rous in 1909. Michael Bishop, Harold Varmus and their colleagues in 1975 discovered that genomes of all normal cells carry DNA sequences that are closely related to viral oncogenes. These cellular genes are termed as protoncogenes. THey are blameworthy for basic cellular functions of normal cells but when mutated they become oncogenes and produce cancer. Many oncogenes have been pinpointed by experiments in which selectted fragments of DNA are added to cells in a culture.

Tumour suppressor genes are more difficultly discerned than oncogenes as they inhibit cancer and are reccessive in action. One of the first tumour suppressor gene to be spotted out was that of retinoblastoma in 1985 by Raymond White and Webster Cavenne.

Alteration In Stucture And Number Of Chromosome Also Cause Cancer

Most tumours possess mutations. It is now clear that mutations in chromosomes appear to be both cause and be a result of cancer. At least three kinds of chromosome rearrangements- deletions, inversions and trans locations may be associated with cancer. Deletions may result in loss of one or more tumour suppressor genes. Inversions and trans locations may result in disruption of functions tumour suppressor genes and generation of fused proteins that may stimulate symptoms of cancer. Fusion proteins are generally formed in myelogenous leukemia, a form of leukemia affecting bone marrow cells. A third process by which cancer may arise due to chromosomal rearrangement is by the transfer of a potential cancer causing gene to a new location where it is activated by regulatory sequences, Burkitt lymphoma is common example.

Viruses Also Cause Cancer

About 95% of the women with cervical cancer are infected with human papiloma viruses (HPVs). Similarly, infection with the virus that causes hepatitis B increases the risk of liver cancer. Epstein-Barr virus causes mononucleosis embracing Burkitt's lymphoma. There are only few retroviruses that cause cancer in humans. Other human cancers are associated with DNA viruses which like retroviruses integrate into the host chromosome but disparate retroviruses donot reverse transcription.

Changes In DNA Methylation Are Often Associated With Cancer

In many cancerous cells the ornamentation of DNA methylation are found to be altered. In some cases, the DNA of cancer cells is over methylated (hypermethylated) or undermethylated (hypomethylated). Hypermethylation is seen to contribute to cancer by silencing the expression of tumour suppressor genes. However, hypomethylation also contributes to cancer requires further research. The role of DNA methylation is interesting because unlike other genetic changes DNA methylation is reversible. These types of reversible genetic alterations are called epigenetic processes.

The treatment of cancer is accessible at present inclusive of chemotherapy, bone marrow transplantation, radiotherapy etc. but the question to be 100% free from cancer still preponderates.

"Patient' with different kinds of cancer(s) have been cured by the use of drugs!"

As We Know It, in 1930, "Cancer of the Lung was a Rare Disease... in the 70's a Drastic Change Occurred - Lung Cancer Had Become The Leading Cause Of Death From Cancer Among Males In The United States of America!"

"Scientists Are Hopeful That Many Cancers Will Be Cured By 'Chemo' In The Future!"

An uncontrolled growth and spread of body cells, is often known as "Cancer." Under a microscope, the black dotted cells known as nuclei are identified as cancer-cells. This identity is defined in comparison to healthy living cells that are small (black dots) with a wall-like perimeter surrounding them. The large black-dotted nuclei has no such wall.

These invading cells can occur in all kinds of animals and plant-life alike. Our focus, in this submission is basically a closer-look at cancer, and a-focus-on-humankind and the very real threat to our health and life.

The process of cell division gets out of hand during the cancerous invasion process when cellular modules are continually produced, vastly more than needed. Making matters worse, these unneeded cells continually produce more unneeded (or wanted for that matter) cell tissue. While these new "wild cells" continually divide, they are in the habit of forming larger and larger masses of new tissue... These are identified as tumors.

Not all tumors are harmful or life-threatening. Some of these "tumors" are benign. Albeit, being of no use to the body, they could easily interfere with its normal activities. These type(s) of tumors are usually surrounded by a "skin-like" membrane, limiting its growth, preventing the invading cells from spreading into other regions of the body. The killer-cells, called "malignant," are not contained... They have no walls holding them in - keeping them from spreading into other areas or regions of the body. They invade all normal cellular tissue - they grow and spread rapidly, invading, dominating, and destroying all normal cellular tissue - these monsters are also tumors - THESE MONSTERS ARE CANCER!

Cancer can occur in any kind of living cell. Being that there are many types of "cell tissue" in existence, the human category alone has over one hundred different kinds of cell tissue... so there can be more than one kind of cancer cell(s). In short, "Cancer is not one disease but a large family of diseases!"

The human body is made up of many different types of cellular tissue. Each of these is in turn, made up of or contains many other different kinds of cell tissue. Many of these cells constantly divide, making it possible for the body to make more of itself, explaining why young humans grow; why the body repairs itself; and the replacing of worn-out tissue, etc.

The four major kinds of cancer are called:

"Carcinomas," "Sarcomas," "Leukemias," and "Lymphomas."

Many types of skin cancer(s) can be typed as "Carcinomas" or cancer(s) of the skin. Identified with the skin-like linings of the lungs, the stomach, internal organs, glands and/or the upper and lower intestines of humans and animals alike.

The connective tissue(s) like bone, cartillage, and fat is attacked by a cancer known as "Sarcoma."

This is the type of cancer that attacked my nine year old niece.

Cancers involving bone marrow cells are "Leukemia."

"Lymphoma(s)" is identified as cancer that attacks the blood. Albeit, both of these cancers attack blood cells, lymphoma is the cancer that attacks the "Lymphatic System" (or Lymph Glands). The lymph is the fluid that fills the spaces between the body's cells.

According to cancer research, more than ninety percent of cancers appear or occur in persons over the age of forty. Due to the fact of people living longer, cancer has become a common disease. This conclusion is partly drawn on the fact that people were not living long lives, primarily past the age of thirty-five or forty.

Chemicals is another factor that is partly to blame for the epidemic. Cigarette smoke being the primary principle in infections then and now.

Cancer, in these United States, is known to be a major culprit in death-dealing infections; second only to 'Heart Disease. Current statistics show only a little over one third of recorded cancer patients as being actual survivors. Many patients are and have been treated with radiation, in carefully administered measures of X-Rays, Radioactive Cobalt, Radioactive Isotopes, and/or Chemotherapy (Drug Treatment).

These types of treatment is intended to possibly cure the cancer patient of his or her affliction(s).

The purpose of research by a multitude of clinics and research institutions all over the world, is to prevent new cases of cancer. The detection of the disease in its early stages allow for an early defence; allowing for the implementation of new and improved treatment while finding new ways to prevent and/or cure this killer disease.

The detection of cancer is paramount. The successful treatment of the disease is more than likely; before the spreading process has begun; taken effect once its presence has been announced.

"Karkinus," as defined by the Ancient Greeks, means "Crab" or "Crab-like" because of the crablike spreading of the invading cancer. "Crab-cancer" is what it was called by the ancient Romans. Malignant growth is also spread when the invader is broken off from the original growth. Different parts of the body are invaded by the cancer cells via the blood stream or the lymph vessels. The new colonies of the evil invaders are called "Metastases."

In an essay by "Helena Curtis," and "T. Gerald Delang," of the Sloan-Kettering Institute for Cancer Research, report an observation of "Chimney Sweeps" in 1775, believed that "soot" from chimneys was the cause of cancer. This report was recorded by a London based surgeon named "Percival Pott." He said that chemicals may not be the ultimate cause of cancer but seem to have had an effect on living cells in such a way that cancer(s) develop.

Chemical based food coloring and flavoring used as

preservatives, along with more than four hundred other cancer causing material(s) commonly used in industrial endeavors, have been identified as root sources with the testing of laboratory animals since 1930. Coal Tar was utilized in producing cancerous cells in rabbits by scientists back in nineteen-fifteen. Fifteen years later, more scientists found the chief carcinogen in the coal tar experiment, according to cancer researchers.

The conclusive details have resulted in the industrial communities steps to try and protect the workers who are exposed to coal, tar, soot, asbestos, dyes in other commonly used material(s).

Clear answers are not always present when chemicals are added to our food(s) as flavoring, coloring, or preservative agents. Many governments attempt to make sure that these types of chemicals are not cancer causing carcinogens. One example of chemical bans is "Cyclamates." These are a kind of artificial sweetener commonly used by consumers. There has been plenty of disagreements by government agencies and researches regarding the banning of these types of chemicals. The United States Government has banned the use of cyclamates due to laboratory test-rats.

"Three out of four," say The American Cancer Society. "Lung Cancer Deaths are the result of cigarette smoking." They state "The Death Rate From Lung Cancer Is Ten Times As High Among Cigarette Smokers As Among

Those Who Have Never Smoked. Those who smoke two or more packs of cigarettes per day, the rate is twenty times as high as among non-smokers."

Laboratory results support these findings. Carcinogens are contained within tars on tobacco. Many scientists agree that more research is needed in order to learn about the reasons why people smoke.

Cancer epidemiology is the study of cancer occurrences in different groups of people. One example of this study is the research on lung cancer in smokers and nonsmokers alike.

Cancer often does not always cause pain or show itself during the early stages. Early cancers are almost always detected by doctors during regular (and/or irregular) physical examinations.

Hidden cancer is often revealed through a simple test could save hundreds of thousands of lives every single year. However, no such test exists - there are particular tests that detect particular types of cancer(s). One such test is called "The Papanicolaou Test." This test is used to detect cancer in the womb, particularly the cervix. The "PAP Test" is the commonly known name for detecting cervix cancer. A trained medical professional can almost always, with the use of a microscope, pick out the cancerous cells as opposed to normal cells. Scientist, collectively, have been utilizing this method of cancer detection for many other forms of cancer.

Researchers say many forms of cancer cannot be traced to outside agents as they are forced to seek the cancer causes within the body. Heredity is a major area of concern as living organisms inherit the basic makeup through the passed down cellular tissue(s). Mice in laboratories have been tested and researched regarding this question; supposing something is or was wrong within the cells of the parent - could this be possible, the passing of cancerous cells via generation to generation?

Closely studied lab mice have been bred relating "generation after generation" in an attempt to compare what happens within and to different groups.

Cancer(s) and other cellular tissue have been transplanted from one animal to another, especially those who happen to be or are much like identical twins. The results vary. In some strains, about ninety to one hundred percent of these mice have developed certain types of cancer. In other strains cancer is almost

CHAPTER 3
COMMON TYPES OF CANCER

- Bone Cancer
- Brain Cancer
- Breast Cancer
- Endocrine Cancer
- Gastrointestinal Cancer
- Gynecologic Cancer
- Head & Neck Cancer
- Leukemia
- Lung Cancer
- Lymphoma
- Multiple Myeloma
- Prostate Cancer
- Skin Cancer
- Soft Tissue Sarcoma

Cancer can typically affect every organ of the body and spread the disease by destroying the neighbouring cells. The various cancers are named typically after the place where they originate in the body. For example, Breast cancer is cancer that originates in the cells of the breast. With about more than 100 types of cancer, this class of diseases is divided into five broad categories.

* Cancer that originates in the skin or in the tissues that cover the internal organs is known as Carcinoma.

* Cancer that starts in the bone, fat muscle, cartilage or blood vessels are known as Sarcoma.

* Cancer in the blood forming tissues like the bone marrow is known as Leukaemia. This type of cancer enters the blood stream and spreads to all the parts of the body.

* Cancer that begins in the immune system of the body is known as Lymphoma and Myeloma.

* Cancer in the cells of the brain and spinal cord are known as Central nervous system cancer.

SIGNS and SYMPTOMS

Pain may be an early symptom with some cancers such as bone cancers or testicular cancer.

Long-term constipation, diarrhea, or a change in the size of the stool may be a sign of colon cancer.

Pain with urination, blood in the urine, or a change in bladder function (such as more frequent or less frequent urination) could be related to bladder or prostate cancer.

Skin cancers may bleed and look like sores that do not heal.

A long-lasting sore in the mouth could be an oral cancer and should be dealt with right away, especially in patients who smoke, chew tobacco, or frequently drink alcohol.

Sores on the penis or vagina may either be signs of infection or an early cancer, and should not be overlooked.

Unusual bleeding can happen in either early or advanced cancer.

Blood in the sputum (phlegm) may be a sign of lung cancer.

Blood in the stool (or a dark or black stool) could be a sign of colon or rectal cancer.

Blood in the urine may be a sign of bladder or kidney cancer.

A bloody discharge from the nipple may be a sign of breast cancer.

Many cancers can be felt through the skin, mostly in the breast, testicle, lymph nodes (glands), and the soft tissues of the body. A lump or thickening may be an early or late sign of cancer.

While they commonly have other causes, indigestion or swallowing problems may be a sign of cancer of the esophagus, stomach, or pharynx (throat).

A cough that does not go away may be a sign of lung

cancer.

A cancer may be suspected for a variety of reasons, but the definitive diagnosis of most malignancies must be confirmed by histological examination of the cancerous cells by a pathologist

There are certain risk factors which might lead to cancer development. These are:

- Growing Older
- Tobacco
- Sunlight
- Ionizing radiation
- Certain chemicals and other substances
- Some viruses and bacteria
- Certain hormones
- Family history of cancer
- Alcohol
- Poor diet, lack of physical activity, or being overweight

Most of these risk factors can be avoided, while some others, such as family history, cannot be avoided. Wherever and whenever possible, steps can be taken in staying away from known risk factors.

Keep in mind that:

- Not everything causes cancer.
- Cancer is not caused by an injury, such as a bump or bruise.
- Cancer is not contagious. Although being infected with certain viruses or bacteria may increase the risk of some types of cancer, no one can catch cancer from another person.
- Having one or more risk factors does not mean that you will get cancer. Most people who have risk factors never develop cancer.
- Some people are more sensitive than others to the known risk factors.

Read on for more information about some of the common risk factors for cancer:

Growing Older

Age is an important risk factor for cancer. Most cancers occur in people over the age of 65. But people of all ages, including children, can get cancer, too.

Tobacco

Tobacco use highly increases the risk of getting cancer, either it be directly using the tobacco or being around tobacco smoke (secondhand smoke). Smokers are more likely than nonsmokers to develop cancer of the mouth, the organs related to respiratory system and the digestive system. They also are more likely to develop leukemia - cancer that starts in blood cells.

Quitting tobacco reduces the risk of cancer (though cancer risk is generally lowest among those who have never used tobacco). For those who have already had cancer, quitting reduces the chances of cancer recurrence.

Sunlight

Natural source of Ultraviolet (UV) radiation is the sun. Other sources are sunlamps and tanning booths. It causes early aging of the skin and skin damage that can lead to skin cancer.

Doctors encourage people of all ages to limit their time in the sun and to avoid other sources of UV radiation:

• Try to avoid exposure to the sun between 10 a.m. and 4 p.m.

• Stay in the shade if you have to go outside.

• Cover exposed areas of the body.

• Wear light-colored, loose-fitting clothing, a broad-brimmed hat and sunglasses with lenses that absorb UV.

• Use sunscreen with a SPF of at least 15. They may help prevent skin cancer.

- Stay away from sunlamps and tanning booths. They are no safer than sunlight.

Ionizing Radiation

Ionizing radiation can cause cell damage that leads to cancer. This radiation comes from rays that enter the Earth's atmosphere from outer space, radioactive fallout, radon gas, x-rays, and other sources.

Radioactive fallout comes from accidents at nuclear power plants or from the production, testing, or use of atomic weapons. People exposed to this fallout may have an increased risk of cancer.

Radon is an invisible, odour-less, tasteless radioactive gas. People working in mines may be exposed to radon.

Another common source of radiation is through medical procedures. Doctors use low-dose radiations for x-rays and high-dose radiations for radiation therapy to treat cancer. The risk of cancer from low-dose x-rays is extremely small as compared to radiation therapy. For both, the benefit nearly always outweighs the small risk.

Talk to your doctor or dentist about the need for each x-ray. Also ask for shields to protect parts of the body that are not in the picture.

Certain Chemicals and Other Substances

Studies show that exposure to asbestos, benzene, benzidine, cadmium, nickel, or vinyl chloride in the workplace can cause cancer. People who have exposure to these things in their workplaces - like painters, construction workers, and those in the chemical industry - have an increased risk of cancer.

Always tend to follow instructions and safety tips when handling harmful substances both at work and at home. Also be careful at home when handling pesticides, used engine oil, paint, solvents, and other chemicals.

Some Viruses and Bacteria

Being infected with certain viruses or bacteria may increase the risk of developing cancer:

• Human papillomaviruses (HPVs) is the main cause of cervical cancer along with some other types of cancer.

• Hepatitis B and hepatitis C viruses might develop into liver cancer.

• Human T-cell leukemia/lymphoma virus (HTLV-1) greatly increases the risk of lymphoma and leukemia.

• Human immunodeficiency virus (HIV) - commonly known as AIDS. People having HIV infection have a greater risk of cancer - lymphoma and a rare cancer called Kaposi's sarcoma.

- Epstein-Barr virus (EBV) has been linked to an increased risk of lymphoma.

- Human herpesvirus 8 (HHV8) is a cause of Kaposi's sarcoma.

- Helicobacter pylorican cause stomach ulcers. It also can cause stomach cancer and lymphoma in the stomach lining.

Certain Hormones

In some health issues, doctors recommend hormone therapy. However, studies show that hormone therapy can cause serious side effects: increases the risk of breast cancer, heart attack, stroke, or blood clots.

Family History of Cancer

A normal cell may become a cancer cell after a series of gene changes occur. Some gene changes that increase the risk of cancer are passed from parent to child. These changes are present at birth in all cells of the body.

It is uncommon for cancer to run in a family. However, several cases of the same cancer type in a family may be linked to inherited gene changes, which increase the chance of developing cancers. However, environmental factors may also be involved. But mostly, multiple cases of cancer in a family are just a matter of chance.

Talk to your doctor if you think you may have a pattern of a certain type of cancer in your family. Your doctor may suggest ways to try to reduce your risk of cancer and also may suggest exams for early detection of cancer.

Ask your doctor about genetic testing to check certain inherited gene changes that might increase the chance of developing cancer. But remember, inheriting a gene change does not mean that you will definitely develop cancer. It means that you have an increased chance of developing the disease.

Poor Diet, Lack of Physical Activity, or Being Overweight

People who have a poor diet, do not have enough physical activity, or are overweight may be at increased risk of several types of cancer.

Some causes of cancer, such as smoking, can be controlled. Others, like a person's age or family history, can't be changed.

Causes

Scientists have found many factors that make a person more likely to get hepatocellular liver cancer.

1.Gender

Men are more likely to get liver cancer than are

women. This could be because of the behaviors listed below, such as smoking and alcohol abuse.

There are also some inherited liver diseases that increase the risk of liver cancer.

2. Cirrhosis

Cirrhosis (suh-row-sis) is a disease in which liver cells are damaged and replaced with scar tissue. This can often lead to cancer. In this country, the major causes of liver cirrhosis are alcohol abuse and hepatitis B and C. Another cause is a disease that results in too much iron in the liver.

3. Diabetes

Diabetes can increase the risk of liver cancer. This is more common in diabetics who have other risk factors such as heavy drinking or viral hepatitis.

4. Obesity

Obesity might increase the risk of getting liver cancer.

5. Aflatoxins

These cancer-causing substances are made by a fungus that can contaminate peanuts, wheat, soybeans, groundnuts, corn, and rice. Long-term exposure to aflatoxins can increase the risk of liver cancer. In the United States and Europe, these foods are tested for aflatoxins.

6. Vinyl Chloride and Thorium Dioxide (Thorotrast)

These chemicals are risk factors for several types of

liver cancer. They have become much less important since Thorotrast is no longer used and exposure to vinyl chloride is strictly controlled.

7. Anabolic Steroids

These male hormones are used by some athletes to increase their strength. Long-term use of these can slightly increase the risk of liver cancer.

8. Arsenic

In some parts of the world, drinking water contaminated with arsenic increases the risk of liver cancer. This is a concern in some areas of the United States.

Less Certain Risk Factors for Liver Cancer

Birth Control Pills

Birth control pills may slightly increase the risk of liver cancer. Most of the studies linking birth control pills and cancer involve types of pills that are no longer used. Birth control pills are now made in a different way, and it is not known if they increase liver cancer risk.

Tobacco

Some studies have found a link between smoking and liver cancer, but the extent of this is not known.

➢ Symptoms of Cancer

- Local Symptoms
- Unusual Lumps
- Swelling
- Hemorrhage/Bleeding
- Pain
- Ulcers
- Jaundice
- Systemic Systems
- Weight Loss
- Poor Appetite
- Fatigue

Cachexia (Loss of weight, muscle atrophy, fatigue, weakness, and significant loss of appetite)

- Excessive Sweating
- Night Sweats
- Anemia
- Thrombosis
- Hormonal Changes

The symptoms of cancer are an important factor in the early detection, though some types of cancer do not exhibit any symptoms at all unless they are in the advanced state. Though each type of cancer exhibits different types of symptoms there are few symptoms that are common to most of the cancers. The patient can exhibit a broad spectrum of symptoms which might not be very specific to the type of cancer like fatigue, unintentional weight loss, fever, bowel changes and chronic cough. Pain is most of the times a symptom of cancer in the advanced form. Pain in the lower back can be symptoms of colon or ovarian cancer while shoulder pain can be a symptom of lung cancer. Though stomach pain can be normally caused by many reasons, stomach cancer is also associated with acute stomach pain.

How harmful is the cancer?

The disease cancer claims the lives of millions of people around the world every year. It is dangerous and life-threatening when it develops as tumors and starts spreading around. The cells may move through the body through lymph systems or the blood and can destroy the other healthy cells in the body. Such a process is known invasion and affects other internal organs other than its place of cancerous origin. Such a tumor that grows, invades and spreads destroying other tissues is known as a metastasized tumor and is a very serious condition which is at times beyond treatment levels.

CHAPTER 4
HOW TO PREVENT CANCER

Food: Eat organic produce, especially fruits whose peels are eaten, and avoid red meat. Eat low on the food chain, choosing more fresh produce and grains and less meat.

Cleaning products: Look under the kitchen sink, and avoid using anything that carries a skull and crossbones. Buy baking soda and vinegar instead - they're just as good.

Cellphones: Limit your calls as much as possible, to lower direct microwave penetration to your brain.

Non-stick cookware and stain repellents: Throw out any old, cracked non-stick pans, since the chemical, PFOA, used to make the non-stick coating has been linked to cancer. It is also presernt in stain-resistant clothing, and waterproof fabrics. Rain-proof gear is OK,, but not next to the skin.

Personal care items: Avoid anything that contains parabens - butylparaben, methylparaben - which in some studies have shown estrogenic activity, and which have also been found in human breast tumours. "We have to create political change so young mothers and fathers don't need to be chemists to decide on a shampoo for their baby."

How is Cancer caused?

The disease cancer is majorly an environmental disease where about 90-95% of the scenarios are caused due to factors like lifestyle and environmental conditions. Only about 5-10% of the cases are caused by genetic disorders. The common factors that lead to environmental causes of cancer are tobacco, obesity, infections, radiation and environmental pollutants. These factors affect the basic underlying genetic cell material leading to the disease.

Treatment course of Cancer

The definitive diagnosis of cancer requires clinical examination of the biopsy specimen. Sometimes initial indication of the malignancy can be through symptomatic or by radiographic imaging abnormalities. Once diagnosed, cancer is normally treated by chemotherapy, surgery or radiation or a mixture of two or more methods. Treatment also depends on the types of cancer and the stage in which the disease has progressed. There are many specific treatment methods that are followed based on the type of cancer and medical advancement has bought in many new types of targeted therapies for the specific kind of cancer. The targeted therapy also works on cancerous cells showcasing abnormal behaviour and reduces the damage caused to normal cells.

Once diagnosed, cancer is usually treated with a combination of surgery, chemotherapy and radiotherapy.

Radiation therapy may be used to treat almost every type of solid tumor, including cancers of the brain, breast, cervix, larynx, lung, pancreas, prostate, skin, stomach, uterus, or soft tissue sarcomas.

Most forms of chemotherapy target all rapidly dividing cells and are not specific for cancer cells, although some degree of specificity may come from the inability of many cancer cells to repair DNA damage, while normal cells generally can.

Contemporary methods for generating an immune response against tumours include intravesical BCG immunotherapy for superficial bladder cancer, and use of interferons and other cytokines to induce an immune response in renal cell carcinoma and melanoma patients.

Pain medication, such as morphine and oxycodone, and anti-emetics, drugs to suppress nausea and vomiting, are very commonly used in patients with cancer-related symptoms. transmission and disease.

Over the last few years there has been a considerable amount of research focusing on an imbalance in the body's Redox homeostasis (balance) as a possible factor in the development of cancer. The theory has been postulated that if the Redox signaling system can be brought back into balance this may prove to be a viable therapy. It may well be worthwhile therefore to look at a Cell Signaling supplement as a means of supporting the best possible defense against heart diseases.

Advances in cancer research have made a vaccine designed to prevent cancer available. The vaccine protects against four HPV types, which together cause 70% of cervical cancers and 90% of genital warts.

The consensus on diet and cancer is that obesity increases the risk of developing cancer. The cancer-fighting components of food are also proving to be more numerous and varied than previously understood, so patients are increasingly being advised to consume fresh, unprocessed fruits and vegetables for maximal health benefits.

Cancer treatment is one of the key concepts related to the study of cancer. Understanding the treatment for cancer is very important to treat the tumors with maximum reliability. This also helps in treating the tumors with least damage to the body of the victim and proves advantageous in minimizing the chances of redevelopment of tumor cells.

Understanding cancer treatment

Treatment for cancerous infections is very sensitive and should be taken in the right manner. Taking any unsuitable or unreliable treatment for cancer can be very risky and cause an irreversible damage to the body cells and tissues. Intensity and tenure of treatment for cancer depends on the character and growth of malignant tumors. Tumor cells can be controlled effectively if detected in time. Chances of curing these malignant cells decrease with an increase in the intensity of cancerous infection. Thus, thorough detection and diagnosis of cancer tumors is very important to plan out the right kind of treatment.

Treatment for cancer usually means the efforts taken for diagnosing and treating the abnormal cells. Main aim of the treatment is to kill the malignant cells and prevent them from further infecting the victim's body. When the cancerous cells invade healthy cells and tissues, such normal tissues and cells are forced to behave abnormally due to lack of vital resources like oxygen and blood. Such abnormal behavior can cause severe damage to some of the vital parts of the body if not controlled in time.

Hence, one of the major concerns of the treatment for cancer is to restrict the cancerous cells from metastasizing. It may use some of the harshest medical techniques to curb or kill such cells as their presence cannot be tolerated for too long. Another main purpose of the treatment is to restore strong immune system in the victim's body to make him more resistible to cancer attack in future. This also helps in gaining maximum benefits from the prescribed medication.

Dimensions of cancer treatment

Taking an apt treatment for cancer is very important to eliminate or curb the abnormal cell growth. Origin of the cancerous cells is the most important aspect in planning a proper treatment for cancer. Not all cancers metastasize at the same pace. Some cancers like the ones originating in the bones, head and neck areas, bloodstream, lungs, abdomen, lymph nodes and breast grow at a faster pace as compared to other forms. Also, these forms of cancers contribute to the maximum cancer deaths worldwide and need a severe form of treatment.

Treatment for cancer also depends upon the nature of tumors. Tumors are usually benign or cancerous. Benign tumors are also termed as non-cancerous or pre-cancerous and are generally harmless to the human body. They do not kill or invade normal cells and tissues and restrict themselves to a particular region. They can be controlled easily because of their inability to metastasize. Also, some of the basic forms of treatments like surgery and regular medication are sufficient to control such tumors and they show very less chances to redevelop.

Cancerous tumors are the ones that are actually responsible for cancerous development in the body. These tumors damage the live cells and tissues very badly and do not allow them to function efficiently. Such cells become abnormal over a period of time and accumulate to form a lump or tumor. These cancerous tumors have high chances of recurrence and metastasize very rapidly. Such malignant tumors need a harsh form of treatment as compared to the benign ones and should be treated under thorough medical supervision.

Age, sex and personal or medical history of the disease also matters in prescribing a viable treatment for cancer. Personal habits and physical attributes also play a main role in undergoing cancer cure. Causes and symptoms may vary form person to person and primarily depend on the organ or the area in which the malignant tumors develop.

Cancer Treatment

Common cancer treatments

Treatments for cancer can be of various types and usually depends upon the cancer stage a person is suffering from.

Surgery is the most common and basic kind of treatment. It is very effective for treating benign tumors. It can also reliably treat the cancerous tumors formed in the initial or the first stage of cancer. Surgery is also recommended for treating tumors in the second and third stages of cancer but can be accompanied by some other treatments like chemical and radiation therapy.

Chemotherapy is another important kind of treatment to cure cancerous tumors. It is usually recommended if the cancer has reached an advanced stage. This treatment can also be prescribed in second and third stages of the disease and can be undertaken simultaneously with surgery.

Radiotherapy is the most advanced form of cancer treatment and is usually taken as the last resort for treating malignant tumors. It focuses more on killing the cells and destroying the infected areas instead of treating the tumors individually. Thus, this also leads to a severe damage to the cells and tissues adjacent to the infected areas and causes a permanent damage to the overall body-functioning.

Cancer treatments are usually severe and should be taken after considering the overall ability of the victim to tolerate such treatments. Treating cancer is a continuous process and depends mainly upon the response of cancer patient. The disease can be treated effectively if the patient responds well to the treatment and undergoes minimum side effects.

How can your effectively prevent cancer?

Cancer prevention is easier than cancer treatment. Though there are many factors that can cause cancer, a few simple changes to your lifestyle can help you prevent them. The below are few methods that you can accommodate or follow to ensure prevention or early detection of cancer.

* Avoid direct or indirect form of smoking

* Look out for skin changes and take care to avoid harmful exposure to the sun

* Maintain a healthy diet of natural fruits and vegetables and limit fat contents

* Keep your alcohol intake within limits

* Remember a healthy exercised body keeps out cancer better

* Learn about any genetic disorders in the family and take necessary screenings

* Beware of harmful substances in your work environment

* Follow safe sexual methods

* Obtain regular cancer screening to detect at early stage

Cancer Research is one of the major scientific efforts that is being undertaken to understand the disease better and find possible therapies. There are many national and international cancer institutes that have been established for this purpose. Since 1971, major advancements have been made in the field of molecular biology and cellular biology leading to many new and advanced treatment modes for cancer.

Everyone has cancer cells in their bodies but these cells do not show up in the normal tests until they have multiplied to a few billion. When doctors inform cancer patients that there are no more cancerous cells in their bodies after treatment, it merely means that the tests are unable to detect these cells because they have not reached the detectable size. How to beat cancer is not an impossible task as long as you know the positives and negatives of food and other factors.

Foods to avoid

When a person has cancer, it is a sign that the person has some nutritional deficiencies. It is necessary to change the diet to strengthen the immune system in order to overcome these nutritional deficiencies. Besides increasing health supplements to strengthen the immune system, it is important to starve cancer cells by not feeding them with the following foods.

Dairy products such as milk, cheese and eggs as these cause the body to produce mucus which cancer cells feed on.

Coffee, tea and chocolate should be avoided as these have high a content of caffeine.

Sugar is a cancer-feeder. Sugar substitutes should also be avoided as these contain aspartame which could be just as harmful.

Meat (except fish) causes an acidic environment

Fried foods should be avoided at all costs

Processed foods such as can foods

Diet

As cancer cells thrive in an acidic environment, it is important to have foods that help to put the body into an alkaline state. Such foods include the following.

Fresh vegetables and fruits

Seeds, nuts and whole grains

Chlorella and spirulina are great health foods as they contain abundant phytonutrients

Green tea has cancer fighting properties

Lifestyle

In addition to a strict diet, a change in lifestyle is necessary to beat cancer.

Exercise daily. Aerobics, walking, swimming and gym workouts help to oxygenate the body

Avoid smoking. This will include avoiding places with cigarette smoke

Have enough sleep, and sleep by 11pm the latest

Drink filtered water to avoid toxins and heavy metals in tap water

Avoid using the microwave oven to heat your food in

plastic containers as this releases dioxin from the plastic into your food

Avoid stress, anger and anxiety as these put the body into an acidic environment. In short, be relaxed and happy

You can beat cancer

Cancer is a disease of the mind and spirit. A positive and proactive spirit will help the cancer person to be a survivor. Deep breathing and daily exercises help to get more oxygen into the cells. Remember, cancer cells cannot thrive in an oxygenated environment

CHAPTER 5
UNDERSTANDING COLON AND RECTAL CANCER

Colorectal cancer or colon cancer occurs in the colon or rectum. The colon is the part of the large intestine. The rectum is the passageway that conncets the colon to the anus.

Colon cancer, when discovered early is treatable. Even if it spreads into nearby lymph nodes, surgical treatment followed by chemotherapy is highly effective. In the most difficult cases when cancer has spread to the liver, lungs, or other site treatment can help make surgery options for many, as well as prolonging and adding to one's quality of life. Research is constantly being done to learn more and provide hope for people no matter what stages they are at?

Most colon cancer develops first as polyps, which are abnormal growth inside the colon or rectum that may later become cancerous if not removed. Colorectal cancer is the third most common type of cancer in men and women in all the different countries. Deaths from colorectal cancer have decreased with the use of colonoscopies and fecal outlets blood tests, which check for the blood in the stool.

Colon Cancer

- Colon cancer is a disease in which malignant (cancerous) cells form in the tissue of colon

- Health history can affect the risk of developing colon cancer

- Signs of colon cancer include blood in the stool or a change in the bowel habits

- Tests that examine the colon and rectum are used to detect the diagnose of colon cancer

- Certain factors and prognosis and other treatment options are possible

Colon cancer is a disease in which the malignant cells form in the tissues of the colon. The colon is the part of the body's digestive system. The digestive system removes and processes the nutrients, vitamins, minerals, fats and carbohydrates, and others. From the food can help pass waste material out of the body.

Colon Cancer symptoms

Signs and symptoms of the colon cancer tend not to be specific. The signs and symptoms can occur due to a number of different conditions. When cancer is detected at early stages, it may not have even caused symptoms

Symptoms can vary accordingly to the specific location within the colon where the tumor is located

- Bleeding in the stool
- Dark colored stool
- Change in the stool consistency
- Constipation
- Diarrhea
- Narrow stools

Test that examines the colon and rectal are used to detect and diagnose it

- Physical examination
- Digital colon examination
- Fecal occult blood test
- Examination by barium enema
- Sigmoidoscopy
- Colonoscopy
- Biopsy

Change in the recovery and treatment options

Change in the recovery options depends on the following

- The stages of cancer, whether the cancer is in the inner lining of the colon, or has spread to the lymph nodes or the other places of the body
- Whether cancer has blocked or made a hole in the

colon

- Whether there are any cancer cells left in the surgery or not
- Whether cancer has recurred
- The patient's general health condition

Rectal cancer

- Rectal cancer is a disease in which cancer cells form in the tissue of the rectum
- Age and history can affect the risk of the rectal cancer
- Signs of rectal cancer include a change in the habits or blood in the stool
- Tests that examine the rectum or colon are used to detect and diagnose rectal cancer

Rectal cancer is a disease in which the malignant (cancerous) cells form in the tissue of the rectum

Signs and symptoms of rectal cancer

- Blood in the stool
- Change in the habits-diarrhea, constipation, feeling that the bowel does not empty completely, stool that are narrower or have a different shape than usual
- Abdominal discomfort-frequent gas pains, cramps, and others
- Change in appetite

- Weight loss for no unknown reason
- Feeling very tired

Tests that examine the rectum and colon are used to detect and diagnose rectum cancer

- Physical examination and history
- Digital rectum exam
- Colonoscopy
- Biopsy

Change in recovery and treatment options

- The stage of cancer, whether it affects the inner lining of the rectum only involves the whole rectum or has spread to the lymph nodes, nearby organs, or others places in the body
- Whether the tumor has spread into or through the bowel wall
- Where the cancer is found in the rectum
- Whether the entire tumor can be removed by surgery.

CHAPTER 6
BEAT CANCER & POWER UP YOUR IMMUNE SYSTEM

Today medicine recognizes that a strong immune system is the best opponent to fight cancer. Knowing how to "power up" the immune system can increase vitality, noticeably improve your quality of life, and even save your life.

Although nutrition, diet, supplements, and many alternative approaches are important for maintaining good health while fighting illness and disease; in many cases, these alone are usually not enough to prevent cancer, or win the "battle" against cancer.

What is needed are "power tools" that:

Provide "noticeable" results

Complement and enhance other therapies, or treatments

Offer immune boosting alternatives which are safer than surgery, drugs, radiation, & chemo which weaken, inhibit and destroy the immune system

- ✓ Provide positive results with no negative side effects
- ✓ Provide preventative and strengthening results

- ✓ Supports harmonious total body functions

Based on these, the following three therapies are identified as "power tools" for fighting cancer and most other degenerative illnesses and diseases:

- ✓ Photon Geni Electromedicine
- ✓ PH Balanced Water (strong alkaline)
- ✓ Infrared Heat
- ✓ Photon Geni Electromedicine

The Photon Geni is an electromedicine instrument which represents the culmination of over 50 years of research and development by Ed Skilling, the world leader in this field of medicine.

The Photon Geni electromedicine instrument provides power to the cells of the body which supports healthy cell functions.

It charges and balances cellular energy throughout the entire body, moves and balances all the fluids of the body (especially the lymph system), re-flows the nerve paths of the body and promotes natural regeneration, and naturally strengthens all the systems of the body, most importantly, the immune system.

It is used for all degenerative conditions including reducing the side affects of all other conventional treatments like surgery and drugs.

It is recommended for digestion, elimination,

infections, injuries, stress and cellular regeneration and relaxation. It is safe and easy to use without negative side effects. It is possible to use the Photon Geni while sleeping to gain the most benefit because more use is better for empowering the cells, tissues, organs and systems of the body including the immune system.

Because the Photon Geni works at the cellular level and moves and balances the body's fluids including the lymph system, it is a powerful complement to nutritional supplements and other therapies that support the immune system.

PH Balanced Water (Strong Alkaline)

Cancer begins, thrives and is difficult to control in an acidic terrain of the body. Acid tissues in the body result from acidic foods we eat, toxins in our environment, the production of acids by the body from every-day bodily functions, and ALL water we drink (chemical tests reveal that most bottled waters are all acidic).

Most of us don't drink enough water and the water or beverages that we do drink are all acidic, including most bottled waters. In most cases, changing diet alone is not enough to alkalize the pH balance of the body.

Drinking strong alkaline pH water contributes directly to balancing the acidic states of the body. It also directly and continually promotes better hydration of the cells, improves digestion and elimination, which provides more harmonic balance of power for a healthier body and stronger immune system.

Given the importance of drinking quality alkaline water, it is recommended to use the best quality water machine for making pH balanced water. The very best water machines for making pH balanced water are from Japan as the Japanese have the most experience in this technology. They have been drinking strong pH water for decades and have been experiencing positive health benefits as a result. The Japanese have the lowest incidence of colon cancer and some other cancers than other countries of the world.

Cheaper versions of these most advanced machines from Japan are available as the Chinese and Koreans have duplicated ("knock off") some of the technology and use cheaper components. When it comes to something as critical and life changing as the water we drink every day, many times better quality, is simply better for you. There are many ways to save money in this world, but risking your health and your quality of life should not be one of those ways.

Drinking quality strong pH balanced water is vital to your health and a "power tool" that supports and complements other health therapies dramatically.

Heat/Infrared

Heat is one of the primary enemies of cancer. This is a

power tool of offense and defense against cancer. This is because cancer cells are weaker than normal cells and are more susceptible to destruction from heat.

Not only does heat kill harmful agents and pathogens in the body, but it also helps detoxify the body. Infrared heat penetrates more than 1.5 inches (40 mm) into the body and because the skin is the largest organ of the body, regularly sweating with infrared helps decrease the toxic load of the body and contributes to better health and vitality and longevity.

Infrared heat increases circulation and it helps detoxify the body through the skin which helps all functions of the body.

Some doctors have concluded that a bio-accumulated toxic load in the human body is responsible for all disease not attributable to bacteria, pathogens, or viruses; a bio-accumulated toxic load in the body is a breeding ground for disease and increases the strength of acidic tissues and terrain of the body.

Using an infrared sauna helps all functions of the body. As it helps with detoxing through the skin, it also helps improve digestion and toxic elimination. It is a powerful tool for supporting the immune system and fighting many cancers.

These 3 power tools: 1) Photon Geni, 2) pH balanced water (strong alkaline), & 3) Infrared heat provide noticeable results with no negative side effects. They are all complementary to other therapies and treatments and are preventative therapies as well. They help strengthen the immune system which is the primary system that beats and prevents cancer and other diseases.

CHAPTER 7
ANTIOXIDANTS, ACIDS, ALKALI AND CANCER

The efficacy of acids, bases and antioxidants in cancer therapy is not a myth. It has biochemical basis informed by modern research (SS Kim et al, 2004; Ian F. Robey & Lance A. Nesbit, 2013). The apparent controversy surrounding this subject emanates from poor coordination of research findings.

BEFORE CANCER

First, let me state that the human body will literally rust away like a nail left under the rain over time without inbuilt natural protective mechanisms. To prevent rust or oxidation, most macromolecules essential for human existence are shielded from molecular oxygen or oxygen equivalents with hydrogen molecules (reduction). Oxygen equivalents are those compounds that remove these protective hydrogen molecules from other compounds.

They are also called oxidizing agents. Compounds that restore these hydrogen molecules are called reducing agents. The two most important organic reducing agents in human body are glutathione and ubiquinone, while the two most important oxidizing agents are molecular oxygen and free oxygen radicals.

APOPTOSIS AND GROWTH SUPPRESSOR GENES

The human body cells are normally continuously moving from resting phase, to growth phase and then multiplication phase. This continuous state of growth and multiplication means that any organ can potentially grow to any size, depending on its natural growth rate. By inference all human beings may also grow into giants. It even suggests immortality of human beings.

Thankfully, every cell has an inbuilt apoptotic clock that ensures that it dies after a specified number of days, making room for incoming cells. Thus red blood cells, for instance, are recycled every 120 days. The size and shape of the cells of individual organs are equally limited prior to their date of apoptosis, by growth suppressor genes (notably p53, AP1, NF-kB) located in the nucleus.

Anything that hinders the functions of apoptosis and growth suppressor genes would obviously be expected to unleash uncontrolled growth and multiplication of cells in any organ of the body. This rapid growth of disorganized and poorly differentiated cells is called cancer.

All anti-growth suppression and anti-apoptosis agents

are called carcinogens. They may be chemicals, radiations, biochemical molecules, acids, bases, free radicals, heat, cold, etc. But they all exert their effect by in activating apoptosis gene or growth suppressor gene. They accomplish this by corrupting the gene coding system in such a way that the codes are wrong (missense) or mean nothing (nonsense).

The code is corrupted due to the insertion of the wrong amino acid code into a gene sequence or the excision of the right amino acid code from the sequence. Consequently the t-RNA misreads or miss-senses the expression of the right apoptosis or growth suppressor protein.

TOXINS, FREE RADICALS AND CARCINOGENS

Toxins are basically those compounds whose activities will directly or indirectly lead to human rust and death by causing catabolic or destructive oxidative reactions in body tissues. The high powered toxic tissue oxidizing agents are called free radicals (ROS and RNS), which are basically free ionized oxygen or Nitrogen atoms (O_2- and N_2-)

When a toxin causes a gene altering damage in the nuclear region of a cell (oxidative nuclear damage) it is then known as a carcinogen. As such not all toxins are carcinogen. Aflatoxin (from mold) is not only toxic to liver cells, but ultimately causes liver cancer, making it a carcinogen.

The detoxification process mainly converts lipid soluble toxins into excretable water soluble glucuronides in three steps. In step one the toxins are aggregated and isolated in the specific organs that neutralize them.

Then glucuronic acid is attached to them in the presence of glutathione which the protective hydrogen molecules. (Note that in fighting oxidants hydrogen (non-ionized) carried by reduced NADPH is a friend, while in acid-base balance ionized hydrogen is the enemy).

Free radicals can also contribute to cancer development by inducing genetic mutation through oxidative nuclear damage, or suppress cancer growth by promoting apoptosis. Step three is the excretion of the toxins.

ANTIOXIDANTS

Compounds use to replenish hydrogen molecules in glutathione and other endogenous reductase enzymes are called antioxidants. A lot of these reducing agents occur naturally in fruits and vegetables. Others are available as drug extracts from plants and animals.

Individual antioxidants target different steps of the detox process. This is why balanced nutrition by itself goes a long way to keep our bodies toxin free. The air we breathe, the food we eat, the water we drink, and the environments we live in are all full of toxins, including heavy metals. To survive as human beings, an extensive detoxification mechanism has to exist.

Every body tissue has detox ability, but the liver, gut, and lymphoid tissues and kidneys play the dominant role. Thus most toxins are trapped, neutralized and excreted through feces, urine or bile. Stagnation or obstruction of flow in any of these three organs, generally leads to a toxic state.

Stressors and nutritional insufficiencies that weaken the immune system also contribute to toxic states allowing micro-organisms to multiply and generate additional toxic substances that must be removed.

Successful detoxification requires a lot of energy, which comes from glucose metabolism. Biochemical energy is not measured in Joules, but in ATPs (Adenosine Triphosphate). The metabolic process for converting glucose to ATP is called glycolsis.

During aerobic glycolysis one molecule of glucose combines with two molecules of ADP3- (Adenosine Diphosphate) and two ionic phosphoric acid molecules to yield two ionic ATP4- molecules and two lactate molecules. The ionic ATP4- molecule gives up one Hydrogen proton (H+) to yield one molecule of ionic ADP3-, which is reused in glycolysis.

Under anaerobic (low oxygen) conditions, ATP is generated differently. One molecule, each, of ADP3- and ionic phosphoric acid accumulated from aerobic glycolysis recombine without glucose to form one molecule of ATP4+ and one hydroxyl molecule. Two hydrogen protons combine with two bicarbonates to end up as carbonic acid inside body cells.

TOXIC ACIDOSIS

Glycolsis can be aerobic when it consumes molecular oxygen, or anaerobic when it consumes oxidizing agents. Both the detox reactions and glycolsis are driven or catalyzed by enzymes, which depend on the availability of specific micro-molecules, proteins, amino acids and vitamins as cofactors for their functions.

By the time enough ATP is generated to keep the body toxin safe, enough carbonic acid hydration of respiratory carbon dioxide (CO_2) has accumulated to keep the inside of every cell perpetually acidic. In a highly toxic state, which includes rapid proliferation of cells, this intracellular acid builds up exponentially beyond survivable limits.

Cancer cells are known to rapidly outgrow their blood supplies and go into severe hypoxic states. This is why the cancer cell nucleus has to rapidly increase the expression of sodium driven proton extruding proteins and enzyme proteins through nuclear sensing of sharp rise in HIF.

Thus, by default, the Intracellular fluid (ECF) of every cell is acidic (low pH) while that of the extracellular fluid (ECF) is alkaline (high pH). It is important to note at this point that while intracellular fluids exist in compartments inside the cells, extracellular fluids coalesce to form a pool in which all body cells submerged.

This ECF pool is represented by intercellular fluid, lymph, blood, and glandular secretions, all of which feed into the circulatory system of the body. ECF acid or base build up in any part of the body is ultimately dissipated into the circulatory system, which centrally maintains a mildly basic pH of 7.20 -7.40.

In addition to mobilizing ammonium and bicarbonate ions the central buffer system has the ability to move chloride ions in and out cells (chloride shift) to maintain acid-base balance.

CHAPTER 8
MEMBRANE SENSORS AND TRANSPORTERS

To keep intracellular acidity below lethal level, the inner surface of the cell membrane has acid sensors and transporters that detect abnormal rise in intracellular acidity and trigger increased extrusion of hydrogen and retention of alkaline bicarbonate ions.

This trigger is mediated by the rise in the blood level of hypoxia induced factors (HIF) and probably acidosis induced factors (AIF). On detecting this rise in HIF, the nucleus temporarily increases the expression of Na-driven proton transport proteins and histidine rich basic proteins.

The ammonium radicals on the amino acids of these basic proteins (especially histidine) serve as physiologic buffers for organic acids.

"Protonation and de-protonation has been experimentally shown to change protein structure and thus, alter protein-protein binding affinity, change protein stability, modify protein function, and alter subcellular localization (Schonichen et al., 2013b).

Evolutionarily, histidines must confer some selective advantage for cancers, as 15% of the 2000 identified somatic mutations in cancer involve histidine substitutions, with Arg-to-His being the most frequent (Kan et al., 2010)".

The nucleus also temporarily steps up the expression of important enzyme proteins that catalyze the buffer reactions, namely mono-carboxylate, carbonic anhydrase, and aminotransferase enzymes.

In a similar manner the external surface of the cell also has alkaline sensors made up of G-protein coupled surface receptors, which also communicate with the nucleus to increase or decrease the expression of relevant proteins and enzymes. As tissue hypoxia decreases, the level of HIF decreases along with nuclear expression of proton extrusion proteins and enzymes.

Failure of this return to normalcy has been observed as one of the hallmarks of early cancer. What started out as a normal adaptive change becomes persistent because of irreversible genetic modifications that triggered it.

CELLULAR SURFACE ACID/BASE REVERSAL

The central physiological buffer system has a maximum capacity to neutralize up to 30 micromoles of acid/gram tissue/min in systemic acidosis or 5-10 micromoles of base in alkalosis.

Beyond these levels, normal body cells are unable to

continue their buffer functions because the enzymes are deactivated. At this point there is a reversal of the normal acid-base distribution on either side of the cell membrane, which is lethal to normal issues. In some critical situations, chloride ions are shifted massively into all body cells (chloride shift) to urgently dilute the extracellular acidity.

But the gastric cells have the natural ability to survive in the presence of high extracellular acidity (HCl at pH of 6.6). How they manage this high extracellular acidity then becomes very important in understanding how cancer cells survive high extracellular acidity with normal intracellular acidity for their survival and proliferation. Some cancer cells are known to have accumulated genetic adaptations that enable them to survive extreme pH conditions (carbonic acid at pH of 6.6).

Gastric cells are shielded from concentrated HCl secreted into the stomach mainly by structural barriers (thick basement membrane, thick mucosal layer and thick mucous layer). There are no natural inhibitors of hydrogen potassium ATPase enzyme that catalyzes the final phase of acid excretion.

In severe cases of Peptic Ulcer Disease (PUD), Gastro-esophageal reflux (GERD), or Zollinger-Ellison Syndrome, when this natural barrier is ulcerated by concentrated HCl, some gastric lining cells undergo goblet intestinal metaplasia (transformation into ectopic intestinal epithelium in the stomach) to secrete neutralizing alkaline fluids into the stomach.

While there is no natural attempt to control the hydrogen potassium ATPase enzymes, pharmacological intervention with proton pump inhibitors (PPIs) like omeprazole has been successful in reducing gastric secretion in severe cases of chronic gastric hyperacidity.

Similarly some esophageal epithelial cells undergo gastric metaplasia to become gastric cells in the face of chronic exposure to reflux gastric acid (Barrett's Esophagus). Acquisition of this missing ability to control hydrogen potassium ATPase and sodium driven proton extrusion by monocarboxylate enzyme appear to be critical to the survival of cancer cells

CHAPTER 9
IN EARLY CANCER

It is important to note that the natural response to extracellular hyperacidity in the GIT depends on the stage and localization of the acidity. Both goblet metaplasia and gastric metaplasia have been recognized as precancerous lesions (carcinoma in situs). At the early stage of Barret esophagus, the response is only structural to prevent cell wall damage.

But when the barrier has failed in the stomach, the response is alkaline secretion. A person on preventive alkaline water will be helping to neutralize the added hypoxic acidity of early cancer in Barret's Esophagus and chronic PUD, but not in any way preventing the occurrence of cancer itself, since proton extrusion in cancer is irreversible.

Any cancer caught at the in situ stage is usually best treated with surgical excision and radiotherapy, rather than alkaline water. The question then is: "Why did prophylactic alkaline water not prevent the metaplasia?"

The answer to that is that while oral alkali intake may cap out at micromoles of alkali per gram tissue, cancer proton extrusion acid build up ranges in nanomoles per gram tissue (a thousand times more). Also intracellular hypoxia and hyperacidity are not the only risk factors for cancer.

Radiations are known to be commonly responsible for skin cancers, even as HPV is known to be responsible for cervical cancer. Prophylactic alkalosis has not been reported to prevent any of them. Sticking to the hype that alkaline water is the best way to prevent and even cure cancer, puts people at risk of missing early opportunities to truly cure cancer.

Alkaline water intake will help the body maximize the physiological adaptive response acidosis. Unfortunately, even at maximum physiological capacity, extracellular buffers are no match for cancer intracellular proton extruders.

As the well adapted cancer cells grow and multiply freely their neighboring non-cancerous cells are rapidly destroyed by ECF hyperacidity creating more space for them to occupy. Thus cancer invasiveness has been shown to correlate with the degree of acid-base reversal across the cancer cell membrane.

At the advanced stage of cancer with ECF acidity readings in nanomols compared to orally boosted alkalinity readings in micromoles, buffer therapy has been shown to be resisted by cancer cells. One such reported example is the inefficacy of a basic drug doxorubicin used in the treatment of Leukemias and lymphomas.

Going by what has been discussed so far, it is obvious

that externally sourced acids and alkali cannot be safely loaded to outweigh tumor generated levels in ECF and ICF. It is also understandable that no single pH balancing agent, can be used to treat both acid sensing and alkaline sensing cancers.

Preventive or prophylactic intake of acidic or alkaline liquids or foods remain relevant only within the physiological buffering range, when adaptive changes are still reversible. Unfortunately at that point the tumor generated acidity would have risen to resistant levels. Preventive alkaline water intake in a person with undiagnosed acid sensing cancer is not likely to retard the growth of the tumor.

Similarly preventive intake of alkaline water in a patient with undiagnosed alkaline sensing cancer will encourage it to grow and establish faster. Patients receiving treatment for emesis gravid arum (vomiting in pregnancy) for instance, cannot be on preventive alkaline regimens in the face of systemic alkalosis from heavy loss of gastric acid through vomiting.

However, it is possible that some people are unable to fully optimize the natural buffer system, due to genetic predisposition or problems related to amino acid metabolism. In such situations, preventive acid or base intake supplements the patients effort to achieve maximum physiological buffering. This can easily account for some of the spectacular results observed in some patients whose cancers were caught early.

the management of cancer remains complicated. When there is a strong family history or occupational predisposition for cancer, cancer screening needs to be done early to search for risk factors and genetic markers.

Where there are suggestions of cancer predisposition, full blood tests, scans, biopsies, endocrinological tests, and radiological test should be done by a primary care provider and reviewed by a team of experts in radiology, hematology, pathology, oncology surgical oncology, gastroenterology, and international medicine.

The apparent controversy surrounding this subject emanates from poor coordination of research findings.

Ketogenic Diet And Hyperbaric Oxygen Therapy On Metastatic Cancer

Gone are the days when cancer meant the end of your world. With science and medical technology booming like never before it is time to bid goodbye to cancer and breathe life in a new way afresh. Well, it is important for us to know that cancer in its various forms can be treated as per the diagnosis. And if you want to find out the perfect balance between a couple of treatments to cure cancer then you have come to the right spot. This article shall focus on fighting metastatic cancer and this is going to be your one stop spot for the solution that you have been looking for across the web.

Metastatic Cancer?

Metastatic cancer is any form of cancer that spreads in various parts of the body. For a clearer understanding of this type of cancer let us take the help of an example, if a person is diagnosed with breast cancer but it spreads to the lungs as well so it takes the shape of metastatic breast cancer and not lung cancer as is the most common confusion among people. The good news is metastatic cancer can be treated with the help of medical progression but the unfortunate part is not all types of metastatic cancer can be treated. Without any further ado let us now find out the treatment that medical science has been able to provide to us.

The treatment

The treatment for metastatic cancer is a careful balance between the ketogenic diet and the hyperbaric oxygen therapy. The ability to be able to strike the right balance between these two treatments is the key to successfully fighting metastatic cancer. This article will provide you with facts as to how both ketogenic diet and oxygen hyperbaric therapy works following that will be the case histories that have proved time and again with desired results.

The Ketogenic Diet

This diet has been a monster hit to fight the advanced stages of metastatic cancer when the cancer bug has spread beyond the original point to other parts. How does it work? This diet is high on fat so much so that the ratio is something as four grams of fat to one gram of carbohydrate or protein. Usually a person's diet is high on carbs and proteins and carbohydrates are burnt into glucose which the cancer cells engulf. Thus following a ketogenic diet helps the person have food high on fat which makes the cancer cells starve to death eventually leading to their death.

Let us now study a few case histories to see the silver lining behind the dark clouds of metastatic cancer. The first metastatic cancer case popped up in the Journal of the American College of Nutrition way back in 1995. This form of diet was experimented upon two children suffering from brain cancer. As luck would have it, they were part of several life threatening chemo and radiation until they were given the ketogenic diet only to see remarkable results. The ketogenic diet is believed to be one of the most conspicuous treatments for metastatic cancer of today.

The Hyperbaric Oxygen Therapy

A piece of news doing the rounds last year stated that

hyperbaric oxygen might be the cause for increasing chances of cancer. The apprehension of many was that the cancer tissue might expand and the heavy flow of hyperbaric oxygen might increase the recurrence of cancer. Extensive studies and experiments have proved that hyperbaric oxygen therapies is an aggressively good treatment in curbing down metastatic cancer and has developed rapidly in the 21st century in the field of nursing and medicine. Much to the surprise of everyone, systematic studies on hyperbaric oxygen therapy has brought to light the fact that it definitely does not enhance cancer but it destroys certain cancer cells from the various subtypes of cancer that prevails. This form of therapy reverses the effects of cancer leading to the death of the cancer cells in case of few of the subtypes.

The right balance

The balance of these two treatments combined in the right proportion helps in curing cancer to the extent of even destroying the traits in the form of cancer cells. If you are still wondering the trick of these two treatments merged together then let me tell you that these two treatments are non-toxic protecting the healthy tissues and in its due course destroying the cancer cells. This statement has been put to experiment with successful results.

CHAPTER 10
BEATING CANCER WITH NATURAL FOOD THAT SUPPORTS LIFE

For over 50 years now, the world has been living in the anxiety of the deadly monster, Cancer. Every day, over 20,000 people die of cancer and with such statistics, it's totally okay for people to be scared. However, there's one pungent remedy that has proved to suppress the fear effectively: knowledge. Doctors and scientists believe that if cancer victims can beat the illness in their minds, then they can beat it out of their bodies. Health magazines, television shows and online blogs dedicated to spreading awareness on the possible antidotes of cancer have been set up and maybe soon enough, these efforts might just pay off.

Nevertheless, orthodox methods to fight cancer continue to go belly up, even with the billions of dollars poured into the research. Chemotherapy seems to be at the top of the, perhaps, current breakthrough but the world is heavily hedging its bets on whether chemotherapy is, indeed a cancer cure or just another risky provisional treatment procedure. Sure there are some patients who have been declared cancer-free after undergoing chemotherapy. But a good percentage of the population has also been reported to be ailing after several years of being diagnosed cancer-free. In addition, the side effects of the procedure have proven quite fatal for some victims, with extreme cases of death been recorded.

So is there a cancer remedy out there that works, without necessarily harming the body? Well, guys like Howard Hoxey, Dr. Max Gerson, and Dr. Johanna Budwig have developed therapeutic formulas that they believe can supply the body with the right metabolic requirements and effectively slow down cancer. And just to be clear, this is not a campaign or claim that this is the definite course of action for cancer cure. I'm just merely stating that I strongly believe that these natural physiotherapies may go a long way to suppress the cancer cells, either alone or in unification with other conventional methods. Here is an all-inclusive approach to curing cancer.

Nutritional treatment

You are what you eat. A proper diet is the backbone of any successful therapy, artificial or not. Scientists believe that certain nutrients such as sugar feeds favor the growth and multiplication of cancerous cells and by avoiding such foods, tumor growth can be slowed down. Other nutrients that should be eschewed include processed foods, coffee, alcohol, fluorides and soft beverages.

Knowing what to eat is crucial for any cancer patient. Herbs, fruits, and vegetables that are highly rich in vitamins are incredible for bodily repair and cleansing. So incorporating foods like broccoli, cabbage, berries, grapes, ginger, garlic, green tea, turmeric and leafy vegetables in your diet will do you some good by providing the necessary nutritional protection.

Cancer patients should be ready to embrace a raw diet, at least until their bodies stabilize. Keeping their fat intake to a minimum is vital. If possible, the use of natural oils like coconut oil is highly recommended. Avocados and nuts may be a good compromise to provide the essential fatty acids in the body necessary for oxygenation of the cells. Above all, digestion should never be knotty. The cancer cells are already straining the body enough and eating heavy foods like sugar, gluten, animal protein and lots of fats will only make the process worse, and probably accelerate tumor growth. Opting for natural supplements that neutralize the acidity in the body and provide an ample supply of systemic and digestive enzymes is therefore obligatory to aid in the cancer healing process.

Immune building and Homeopathy

The body naturally depends on its own immunity provided by the white blood cells, and I believe this was the original plan up until genetic disorders became a thing. Bearing in mind that cancer cells heavily mutate once in the body, it is possible for the body, by virtue of innate immune intelligence, to defend itself against this multiplication before it becomes uncontrollable. A special group of white blood cells whose sole purpose is to attack and destroy abnormal cells through the lymphatic system exists. The key now lies in energizing these special cells. Dietary supplements such as Aloe Vera and mushroom extracts are ideal in this case.

Again, in homeopathy, the body's natural healing power is believed to be activated. Here, small dosages of remedial substances are given to the patient to boost the immunity. Though research on homeopathy is still fragmentary, it is possible that it may prove counteractive in the near future.

Detoxification

Accumulation of metabolic wastes in the body accelerates tumor multiplication. For effective cancer healing, it is important to flush out the accumulated wastes and toxins from the body. Lots of resources that offer knowledge on body cleansing can be found online and in books. Body purification reduces the load on the liver and kidneys, stimulating the immune system to fight the cancerous cells wholly. To speed up the detoxification process, there are additional lifestyle practices that can be adopted at home as an addendum. Frequent exercising and stretching ensure that the white blood cells in the body remain active throughout. Taking regular baths and drenching in a sauna every now and then keeps the skin clear to allow for reclamation through sweat. Fasting rejuvenates the body and foods like coffee enemas and castor oil prevent the reabsorption of toxins.

Raw chemotherapy

Artificial chemotherapy for cancer cure, though feasible, can have adverse secondary effects like hair loss and body weakness among others. What most people don't know is that there are risk-free chemotherapies that effectively prevent malignancy in the body. Naturally occurring foods like apricots seeds and apple pits contain Amygdalin that actively targets and destroys the tumor. Other supplements like shark cartilage and liver oil cut off blood supply to the cancerous cells. Of course, these treatments are not entirely standalone and are often applied as part of the comprehensive cancer therapy.

All in all, embracing a more body-friendly lifestyle is the most imperative part of this natural therapeutic process. Taking regular naps to the fullest allows the body to rebuild and purify itself from carcinogens that build up in the body while you're awake. Exercising frequently and basking in the sun for vitamin D are all part of the salutary regime that you should aspire to adopt. Slowly, your body rebuilds its immunity and fights the cancerous cells, one step at a time.

We all know how it is, a person hit with a cancer diagnosis is initially lost and scared, not knowing where to start or where to apply the brakes. If you find yourself in such a situation all you need is a road map for taking full control of your health and how to combat the illness.

The truth and the gospel truth is that when situation are bad health-wise, decision to live or not to live, to survive or not to survive is yours and yours alone no one can take that decision for you, and it is the intensity of that decision that propels you to desperately search for solutions.

A situation by which someone surrenders his or her life to experimentation is sheer madness, for the sake of emphasis decisions bother my on your health need to be effectively taken by you, no one, 1 repeat nobody is qualified to take rush decisions for you, not even your surgeon or your oncologist.

You are the beauty of God and you are unique, because of that uniqueness in you the decision on what to do fight disease is yours and yours alone.

The aim of this write up is to help and to ginger you make informed decisions based on informed choices, period. I have the privilege of introducing to you the book "Beating Cancer with Nutrition"

Whether you are in the last stage, early stage of your

cancer, or a medical or alternative practitioner or a care giveror health professionals in general, " The book,"Beating Cancer with Nutrition"explains in detail everything a cancer patient need to know about diet, lifestyle and specific dietary supplements to boost the immune system and to selectively kill cancer cells.

Do you know that 40 percent of cancer patients die from malnutrition and not cancer itself.The author stress that the underlying condition of the disease need to be addressed first.

What is the key to beating cancer with nutrition? You will find out in the book, proper. A tip of the iceberg good nutrition, attitude, exercise and detoxification of essential organs such as the liver must are all necessary.

Do you know that tumors are enormous sugar absorbers? Yes, when you eat too much sugar in the diet even natural sugars, cancer spreads easily. Why? Because the walls of the capillaries become permeable and the tumors spread through the cell wall.

Cancer patients should avoid foods containing processed sugar, cancer spreads as a result of lack of oxygen, immune suppression, sugar feeding and toxin overload. For a start, cancer patients should avoid foods containing processed sugars and practise breathing from the diaphragm.The author advocates aggressive nutrition which leads to bolster the immune system. He also suggested vitamin supplements and specific recipes which contain the essential cancer fighting nutrients.

Today food is big business, farmers and manufactures will add anything that is legally allowed to enhance their product to maximise profit. This is typical of the food we are now eating. Supermarkets have taken over the supply of our food and most of what we eat is no longer fresh and has often been in storage for many months. What we are eating today is so processed that our meals are nutritional deprived.

To maintain our health and keep us free of diseases we have to feed every cell in our body and we do that with natural food that's been designed to support life. Food is our medicine we take daily to keep us healthy and disease free because it builds up our immune system and makes us resilient to all ailments from colds and the flu right through to heart disease and cancer.

Natural food is food in its natural state which has been grown in the ground and arrived in our shops directly from a farm and not via a factory. Natural food is full of vitamins, minerals and phytochemicals which the human body needs to maintain health. There are some foods that are classed as super foods or healing food because of their ability to fight diseases to help us regain our health.

There are three vitamins that are essential for anyone to stay free of cancer and they are vitamin A, C and E. There are many foods with these vitamins but are easily gained by eating fresh oranges, avocados, kiwi fruit and berries. It is well known that when a certain food is processed it looses many of the compounds that are helpful.

Other beneficial foods are tomatoes which contain lycopene and are helpful for both prostate and breast cancer patients. Watermelons are full of antioxidants which are known to prevent the formation of free radicals that causes cancer. Lettuces are full of fibre which we need and one of the best foods for a cancer patient is those from the cruciferous family which are broccoli, cauliflower, brussel sprouts, cabbage and spinach.

Other important foods are members of the onion family which include leeks, chives, shallots and especially garlic. Onions are literally packed with valuable compounds and are also full of antioxidants. The more pungent an onion tastes and smells the higher the antioxidant value. Onions are also rich in sulphur compounds and it has been regarded as a cancer fighting nutrient. High onion consumption is thought to be the main reason why there is a lower risk of bowel cancer.

Dietary antioxidants which we obtain from these foods are the foundation of cancer prevention and must be consumed on regular bases from a variety of fresh produce. Our western health care system does not have the answers to cancer with their toxic treatments but nature does through the many foods it produces.

Cancer Fighting Foods

Cancer cells are always present in the body and are normally kept in check by our body's own natural defense system. Do you know how the body's natural defense system works and where it gets the ammunition to do so? Do you know at what point the body succumbs to the disease named cancer?

Millions of cancer cells are present in the body from time to time. However, when the cancer cell count reaches the billions, we know the body's natural defense system is not working. Cancer cells seem go undetected as foreign cells by the body. Since cancer cells grow more quickly than normal cells they can replace healthy cells almost unnoticed by the body until we feel something is wrong, a tumor, or an organ is malfunctioning.

Cancer has occurred in your body over a long period of time due to many different forces. Outside influences such as environment, exposure to toxins, smoking, second-hand smoke, tremendous shock, and cancer-causing foods can and do cause cancer.

However, cancer can be cured. Studies have proven that a nutritious diet of anti-oxidant foods and nutrients can cure cancer. Cancer fighting foods are as close as your local grocery store shelves. All you need is the knowledge of which particular foods and the correct recipes and you will be able to cure your cancer condition naturally. In this case, knowledge is the power to heal.

A wide variety of foods makes a lifetime cancer-free diet. There is a process to learning how to make food selections and cook in a way that not only cures cancer, but prevents the disease from permeating your body. Two-time cancer survivor and author Carol Patterson has developed many wonderful tasting recipes using cancer fighting foods. Her second diagnosis of cancer prompted the doctors to suggest radical surgery. The author chose alternative cancer cures to save her body from being disfigured and horrendous exposure to chemotherapy again.

The cancer fighting foods program works and be assured that your cancer can be cured. Cancer cures are as close as the local grocery store or health food market coupled with the correct recipes and you will be able to cure yourself of cancer and to maintain a healthy body for the rest of your life. The National Cancer Institute estimates that roughly one-third of all cancer deaths may be diet related. What you eat can hurt you. On the other hand, what you eat can also help you. Knowing which foods are cancer fighting foods, and making the correct choices can save your life.

Many of the common foods found in grocery stores or organic markets contain cancer fighting anti-oxidants and can cure cancer naturally. The antioxidants neutralize damage caused by cancer-causing free radicals and change them into phytochemicals which battle cancer cells. Scientists are just beginning to explore this amazing phenomenon.

Worldwide, we are beginning to realize that the modernization of our food processing system in the last 50 years has led to almost epidemic proportions of cancer and heart disease. Not only are these foods contributing to an enormous obesity problem because of chemical ingestion, but processed foods are poisoning our bodies one day at a time. Over a period of 25-40 years, major damage has been done to our bodies by eating chemically processed foods; and the result is deadly cancer and heart disease.

The good news is that the body has extremely resilient recuperative abilities. Cells divide and regenerate daily, including cancer cells. Cancer cells are missing two essential amino acids: Linolenic Acid and Linoleic Acid. That being the case, it is very logical to realize if we feed the cancer cells the missing amino acids and nutrients, the cells will have the ability to morph and regenerate themselves into healthy cells. The concept is quite simplistic, but it works. Cancer can be cured and many people have been cured from cancer with this concept using cancer-fighting foods.

What researchers are finding is we are what we eat!

All over the world, our diet has changed from the times when we ate mainly farm-fresh foods. We go to the grocery store and buy many processed foods which have chemical preservatives and are generally not healthy for us. In many cases, these foods actually cause cancer one day at a time over a period of years.

On the other hand, there are many foods in our grocery stores which have natural antioxidants and the ability to fight off cancer as well as maintain normal body health. Once you know the correct cancer fighting foods, you can institute a natural cancer cure.

The National Cancer Institute recognizes that diet and nutrition play a big part in fighting cancer. They recommend eating at least five daily servings of fruit and vegetables as part of a low-fat, high fiber diet. Many cancer fighting foods which are high in anti-oxidants are nuts, fruits, and vegetables.

In general, in the western world, our daily diet today is out of balance. We eat too much food; we eat too much meat and fat; we eat too much sugar and salt, and our diet lacks fruits, vegetables, nuts, and grains. Our normal daily diets are comprised mostly of up to 45% fats. A healthy fat intake should be 30% or less of the total day's food intake.

The National Cancer Institute states that diet and nutrition are factors in 60% of cancers in women and 40% of cancers in men.

Today more and more studies are proving that we can beat cancer with the ammunition of nutritious foods and a balanced diet. John's Hopkins University in their cancer studies has a new update verifying these studies.

It has become common knowledge that nutritional food intake is essential to fighting cancer. It is not logical that the reverse could be true? The wrong foods can and do cause cancer. Not too difficult to figure out!

The National Cancer Institute and the Federal Food and Drug Administration agree that Americans should eat more fiber and reduce their fat intake. These authorities also stress that the freshness of food is an important factor.

Fresh foods straight from your own garden or the farm stand would be the best cancer fighting foods, plus they are delicious tasting! When you use fresh foods for your meals, and prepare them yourself, you know what you are eating. This is essential to a creating a cure for cancer for yourself or loved one.

There are numerous published reports documenting the healing qualities of a healthy diet. The idea of consuming fruits and vegetables while they are still in their natural state means that we preserve the natural nutrients to put into our body.

When making juice from fruits or vegetables, drink the juice within five minutes of processing to preserve the natural nutrients.

Once the principles of fresh food make sense to you,

the idea of store-bought, processed food reveals itself as a large part of the problem. Learn to look at the labels on the back of food packages. The best advice is to eat food in its natural state as it comes from the grower. If you can grow your own vegetables, that is an even better solution.

You will begin to realize the more modern we have become in terms of our food process; the more we now have epidemic high levels of cancer, heart disease and obesity and increasing year after year. There is a direct correlation of processed foods and disease which scientists are proving daily.

There is something drastically wrong with this picture! People no longer have to be deathly sick with cancer. Cancer can be cured through cancer fighting foods.

Preparing your own fresh juice and food is slightly more work, but consider the alternative. Other countries such as Japan and China do not have the heart disease, obesity or the cancer problems which we have in the western world. Asian foods are mostly vegetable, nut, fruit and fish based. The health problems of heart disease, obesity, and cancer in the western world, and the food differences between our foods and Asian foods have direct correlation.

Medical and scientific resources are now stating the reason for the high spikes in illness throughout the world is because of processed foods. When you hear a food warning, one at a time on a radio show or a morning talk show, it does not have the impact as it does in written reports complied by government agencies and noted authorities.

It is very logical to see: We are what we eat!

Listed below is a chart of FDA approved fruits and vegetables. Make note on this list; there is plenty of food to eat! Making delicious and healthy cancer fighting foods from this listing is not difficult at all.

CHAPTER 11
FDA CONSUMER JOURNAL'S TOP 20 FRUITS, VEGETABLES, AND FISH

TOP20 FRUITS	VEGETAB	FISH
Bananas	potatoes	shrimp
Apples	lettuce	cod
Watermelon	tomatoes	Pollock
Oranges	onions	catfish
Cantaloupe	carrots	scallops
Grapes	celery	salmon
Grapefruit	sweet corn	flounder
Strawberries	broccoli	sole
Peaches	green cabbage	oyster
Pears	cucumbers	orange

		roughy
Nectarines	bell peppers	mackerel
Honeydew melon	cauliflower	ocean perch
Plums	leaf lettuce	rockfish
Avocados	sweet potatoes	whiting
Lemons	mushrooms	clams
Pineapples	green onions	haddock
Tangerines	green beans	blue crab
Sweet cherries	radish	trout
Kiwis	summer squash	halibut
Limes	asparagus	lobster

Many of the foods on both the FDA recommended list and the cancer fighting foods are the same. Take the time to cross-reference this list with the cancer fighting foods list below. You will see that many of the foods are the same. Amazing!

By changing your diet, and going back to the way we ate 30-50 years ago without processed foods in our diet, you will have the ability to make your body strong and healthy again. Processed foods are a no-no. A lifetime of processed foods can lead to cancer, heart disease, and obesity, which have all become epidemic proportion in the western world.

We have gotten away from true center in our food intake.

We eat too much, and especially eat too much of the wrong foods. If you look at the daily diet of an average teenager, think fast-forward 25-40 years from now, to the amount of illness which will strike their lives after 25-40 years of ingesting chemically processed foods. This is one of the reasons childhood obesity is at epidemic levels. These children do not have a chance for a long healthy life unless they change their eating habits and stop eating processed foods and chemicals.

We drink processed soft drinks and orange juice which are filled with high sugar content, we eat processed meat and dairy products which have high chemical content, and we cook our food to the point where we have lost the nutrition either to the water in the boil, or the flame of the cooking process.

Foods, as prepared in most Asian countries, do not

have the cancer risk we have developed over time in our food processing and preparations in the western world.

CANCER FIGHTING FOODS

There is logic to the association of healthy foods and the relationship to a healthy body.

Listed below are foods which are cancer-fighting foods which can be used to cure cancer. These foods also happen to be foods for living a wonderfully healthy lifestyle.

Avocados

Broccoli, cabbage, and cauliflower

Carrots

Chili peppers and jalapenos

Figs

Flax

Garlic

Ginger

Grapefruits

Grapes, red

Green and yellow leafy vegetables

Kale

Licorice root

Mushrooms

Nuts

Oranges and lemons

Papayas

Raspberries

Red wine

Rosemary

Seaweed and other sea vegetables

Sesame Seed Oil

Soy products such as Tofu

Sweet potatoes

Teas: Green Tea and Black Tea

Tomatoes

Turmeric

Turnips

Nature has provided a plethora of foods for us to eat and enjoy a healthy life. Have some fun creating recipes that include the cancer fighting foods in this book. Explore your grocery store in the vegetable and organic sections. There are many foods readily available at your local grocery or health food store on this list.

Cancer is so common, in fact, that in the Unites States alone, "It is estimated that 1,638,910 men and women

(848,170 men and 790,740 women) will be diagnosed with and 577,190 men and women will die of cancer... in 2012."

And in case you didn't know, anyone can get cancer - men, women, old, young, children, women with and without children. Cancer does not discriminate and in fact, according to the American Cancer Society, although childhood cancers are rare, they make up "... less than 1% of all cancers diagnosed each year." Although the percentage amount is small, the person count is still too high since this 1% figure means that about 12,000 children under the age of 15 in the United States alone will be diagnosed with cancer in any one year.

Cancer also affects all parts of the body - brain, eyes, stomach, anus, cervix, breasts, prostate and more. In fact, the American Cancer Association has listed 29 main types of cancers with some having derivatives. The main types of cancer worldwide, though, tend to be lung, stomach, liver, colorectal, breast, and cervical cancer. According to the International Agency for Research, in economically developed countries, the three (3) most commonly diagnosed cancers are:

1. For Men - Prostate, Lung & Bronchus and Colon & Rectum cancer

2. For Women - Breast, Colon & Rectum and Lung & Bronchus cancer

While in developing countries, the three (3) most

commonly diagnosed cancers are:

1. For Men - Lung & Bronchus, Stomach and Liver cancer

2. For Women - Breast, Cervix Uteri and Lung & Bronchus cancer

And there's more! According to WHO, "Deaths from cancer worldwide are projected to continue rising, with an estimated 13.1 million deaths in 2030." That's almost double the current annual amount of cancer deaths. Frightening isn't it?

Well, you already know the old adage, "Prevention is better than cure." That's also so very true when it comes to cancer. You have the power to prevent and protect you and your loved ones from cancer. No expensive equipment or fancy foods are needed. The SOLUTION - Fresh Fruits and Vegetables! Yes, it's that simple!

How Can Fresh Fruits and Vegetables Help in the Prevention of Cancer?

Fresh fruits - as opposed to canned fruits or preserved fruits - are best for fighting and preventing cancer. Fresh Fruits and Vegetables contain lots of Vitamin C as well as nutrients and phytochemicals that act as antioxidants. This mix of Vitamin C, nutrients and antioxidant properties of fresh fruits and vegetables are very important, not only for preventing cancer, as they:

a. Help neutralize free radicals in the body and thus prevent the uncontrolled growth and spread of abnormal cells in the body that can lead to cancerous growths.

b. Prevent clogging of the arteries, so that there is enough oxygen in the blood and there is free and adequate blood flow throughout the body bringing adequate amounts of oxygen and nutrients to all body cells and resulting in reduced risk of developing a heart and other diseases, such as cancer.

c. Prevent premature aging so that skin remains supple not dry and wrinkles are kept to a minimum.

d. Facilitate waste elimination, purification of the blood and the proper functioning of the intestines and digestive system due to their fibre content.

e. Strengthen the immune system as well as bones, teeth, nails and arteries.

How to Incorporate Fresh Fruits and Vegetables in Your Daily Diet

Trying to eat the recommended 5 to 6 servings of fruits and vegetables each day [1 serving is equal to ½ cup] can seem a burdensome task but using these meal tips can ensure that you get it all in:

a. Incorporate a fruit, fruits or some vegetables into breakfast - whether it's a slice of your favourite fruit or a melange of your favourite fruits mixed together in a Smoothie or a delicious Rainbow Vegetable Omelette

b. Snack on a fruit for your 10 o'clock or mid-morning break - one fruit or several individual fruits or a fruit salad incorporating different coloured fruits to take the bore out of eating fruits.

c. Make the salad your main dish during lunch. That's right. If you were to divide your plate into sections mentally, your salad or vegetables should take up at least half (½) of your plate. Don't do like most people and eliminate vegetables from your lunch or put a token spoonful of vegetables on your lunch plate.

d. Instead of ice-cream or cheesecake or pastry for dessert have a serving of fresh fruits or a fruit salad.

e. For your afternoon snack, get rid of the chocolate bar, cheese sticks and potato chips. Again have a fruit or a fruit salad. Choose a different fruit or mix of fruits each time to ensure that you don't get bored and treat eating fruits as a chore.

f. Try a different colour fruit or vegetable each day (red, orange, yellow, green, purple, etc.) or try a rainbow mix of colours each day. Each colour fruit and vegetable provides the body with a different set of nutrients and vitamins.

I have to agree with the famous 19th century, French gastronome, epicure, lawyer and politician - Jean

Anthelme Brillat-Savarin (1755 - 1826) - when he says "Tell me what you eat and I will tell you what you are." If you forget to include or deliberately omit fresh fruits and vegetables from your daily diet, it is sure to manifest itself one day in the form of some type of cancer or illness, blockage of your arteries and premature aging. All of which can be prevented with a few dollars of fresh fruits and vegetables purchased each week as opposed to the thousands of dollars that will be needed to cure your cancer through radiation, chemotherapy, medication, doctor visits, hospital visits and stay.

What Does Water Have to Do With Fresh Fruits, Vegetables and Cancer Prevention?

So you've eaten your 5 to 6 servings of fruits and vegetables for the day. Great! Well what about the water? If you don't drink your daily recommended 6 to 8 glasses of water then you've counteracted all the good that your fruits and vegetables were supposed to do. Why? If you don't drink enough water, you prevent your body from properly eliminating waste and toxins. This resulting build-up of waste and toxins in your body, over time, will lead to cancerous growths in the body and by extension cancer.

Drinking any liquid - sodas, canned or bottled drinks, beer and other alcoholic beverages, milk, tea, coffee - is not a substitute for water. Many people erroneously count their intake of, especially beer, milk and soda, as part of their daily water intake since they argue that they all contain water. Your body knows what it needs - water. Does a man who has spent a considerable amount of time in the dessert ask for milk? No! He asks for water! Does a woman ending a long fast after a few days ask for beer? No! She asks for water! Water, by itself, has alkaline, thirst quenching and purifying properties that soda, milk or beer cannot provide.

If, however, in addition to your daily intake of 5 to 6 servings of fruits and vegetables, you drink the recommended 6 to 8 glasses of water each day, you will be helping to flush toxins and other waste from your body, purify your blood, keep your skin supple, reduce acidity in your body and keep viruses out of your immune system. All pluses for your health.

So eat your 6 servings of fruits and vegetables each day and keep cancer at bay!

CHAPTER 12
FUNDAMENTAL FEATURES OF ORAL HYGIENE

Personal hygiene, which includes oral hygiene and dental care, plays a vital role in every individual. Oral hygiene is the process of keeping your mouth, teeth, and gums clean to prevent tooth and gum diseases such as cavities, gingivitis, periodontal and halitosis disease. Proper hygiene can ward off severe diseases, and also help you achieve optimal health condition as manifested in whiter teeth, pink gums, and fresher breath. Even though a good dentist can work wonders, oral hygiene begins at home. Here are a few helpful tips to improve your daily routines on healthy oral care.

Brushing and flossing

The first and most significant hygiene practice is cleaning your teeth regularly. Brushing your teeth on a daily basis is a practical preventive care as it helps to remove plaque and to hinder the formation of tartar. Always brush your teeth after every meal and before bedtime. Brush two times daily and frequently. Use toothpaste that contains fluoride when brushing, to help prevent cavities. Remember to brush your tongue as well, to get rid of mouth-borne bacteria. Use a soft head toothbrush to avoid causing irritation of the enamel.

Another vital oral hygiene practice is to floss. Flossing each time after brushing helps to remove food debris and plaque stuck in your teeth, and also helps with breath. Floss inner areas of your teeth, and ensure you don't hurt the gums while flossing. You may ask your dentist if you should use dental tap or dental floss. A mouthwash can also help with oral health and help you achieve fresher breath. Make it a habit to gargle after every meal.

Healthy diet

Oral hygiene can be influenced by diet choices and lifestyle. A good diet is necessary for healthy teeth and gums and for overall health. Avoid foods with high concentration of sugar such sweetened teas, soda, and fruit juices. Drinking a lot of water is very important for oral hygiene. Fresh fruits such as apples and also vegetables, grains and chicken can be good for healthy oral hygiene. Acidic foods and drink should be avoided as they can promote enamel wear and tooth decay. Avoid drinking too much red wine, tea and coffee, as they cause teeth staining.

Long term dental care

There are good long-term dental care practices that can prevent frequent dentist visits, gum diseases, yellowing teeth, and awful breath. Replace your toothbrush every 2 months to facilitate proper cleaning. Stop smoking and chewing tobacco. Smoking can bring various effects to your body and oral healthy. Massage your gums after cleaning your teeth to stimulate flow of blood to the gums and enhance gum health. If you have dentures and retainers, it is important to properly clean them, as it is to clean your teeth. Children should start visiting a dentist on a regular basis to help identify any potential problems and begin a lifetime of good oral care.

Visiting the dentist regularly

Regardless of how well you care for your teeth at home, it's still important to visit the dentist regularly. Regular dental checkup is necessary for optimum oral care and hygiene. Get teeth checkups and cleanings at the dentist every six months. Your dentist or oral hygienist has special skills and instruments to clean your teeth more thoroughly and also provide you with important oral care tips. It is very important to have a qualified dentist and also to have good dental insurance that covers your dental treatments.

Practicing good oral health can aid in your overall

wellbeing. These are just a few of the things that can help you maintain good oral hygiene, have a dazzling smile and most importantly, stay healthy.

CHAPTER 13
COMMON ORAL HYGIENE PITFALLS: HOW TO OVERCOME THEM

You wonder why you are brushing your teeth three times a day and perhaps you are also using a mouthwash but you are still occasionally suffering from oral hygiene problems such as bad breath and tooth decay. So what could be the problem? Without your knowing, oral hygiene pitfalls could be slipping their way into your lifestyle. To help you avoid them, here are some of them:

Binge eating

You know what this is. It is those occasional times throughout the day when you take a cup cake, a bar of chocolate, or some cookies and eat them in between meals. This exposes your teeth to food debris because you usually only brush your teeth after major meals such as breakfast, lunch, and dinner but not after binge eating. Limit yourself to scheduled snacks and brush your teeth after which.

Bed snacks

Here is another problem: some foods especially junk foods, candies, and chocolate bars always seem to find their way under your pillow. Especially if you have television inside your room, snacking can be a luxury you want to indulge on. But when you snack inside your room, it is usually not followed by tooth brushing.

Sugary drinks

Even if you have the habit of brushing your teeth after every meal, snack, or binge eating, you are probably not doing so after drinking bottled juices, canned soda, or any other sugary drinks. Well, this is not saying you should because it is ridiculous. Instead, you might want to avoid these drinks. If you want them, you can have them during your meals or snacks.

Old toothbrush

As long as I am brushing my teeth regularly, I should be okay. And there is some truth to that. But the question is how old is the toothbrush? Take note that even your toothbrush has an expiration date. After some time, it will host too many bacteria that it is already counterproductive. It might also lose its brittleness and ability to clean thoroughly. Replace your toothbrush around every 2 to 3 months.

Time rush

It is a nice idea to always have time to brush your teeth after every meal. But that is the problem: time. Especially among businessmen and city employees, they may no longer be afforded this time. Even if they find time to brush their teeth, they no longer do so thoroughly. Make sure that you find time and do proper time management.

Neglecting dentist visits

Another result of the 'As long as I am brushing my teeth regularly, I should be okay' notion is that it makes people neglect visit to the dentist. Take note however that your toothbrush can only clean so much. Buildups will soon develop on your teeth and only your doctor can remove those. Have regular dentist visits and do dental cleaning at least annually.

Mouthing/Biting

If you still have the habit of biting things like the head of the pencil of your pen, it is definitely something you need to overcome. This also includes nail biting and thumb sucking. These habits are bringing unknown bacteria into your mouth and can contribute to poor oral hygiene.

CHAPTER 14
THE PERFECT DIET PLAN: EAT LEAN PROTEIN MEALS AND FORGET THE UNBALANCED DIET

Have you ever been told that high protein diets are bad for you? Maybe you've even heard someone say that high protein will cause kidney damage. It's obvious that the talk of high protein diets is controversial, even with experts. But, we're not talking about "high" protein diets here that eliminate carbohydrates. That is really an unbalanced diet. Actually, we're talking about including healthy portions of lean protein to every meal and snack that includes a healthy portion of carbohydrates and essential fats to make the perfect diet plan. It's important to eat a complete, lean protein with every meal. Though research shows that a higher protein diet is completely safe in healthy individuals and contributes to a healthier body, it is very difficult to get adequate amounts with the three typical meals of the day. To eat lean protein meals at just breakfast, lunch, and dinner is usually not enough. You may have to include a protein with your snack meals too. Besides, eating protein with all meals, including snacks, eliminates the unbalanced diet.

Wondering why protein is so good for the body?

Well, there are many reasons, but these are a few of the healthiest benefits and even maximize fat loss:

Protein is thermogenic and can lead to a higher metabolic rate. It requires 25 to 30 percent of energy for metabolic processing (i.e., digestion, absorption, and assimilation) which is much higher than carbohydrates at 6 to 8 percent and fat at 2 to 3 percent. This means higher fat loss during dieting and less fat gain while overeating.

Protein increases glucagons which is a hormone that fights the effects of insulin. Additionally, it helps decrease the making and storing of fat in adipose and liver cells. This also means higher fat loss during dieting and less fat gain while overeating.

Protein increases IGF-1 which is an anabolic hormone that increases muscle growth. Higher IGF-1 spares muscle while dieting and increases muscle mass while overfeeding.

By increasing protein while decreasing carbohydrates, LDL cholesterol and triglycerides (the bad fats) are lowered while HDL (the good fats) are increased.

Not sure what lean protein sources to include?

Well, look no further. These are the cleanest, or healthiest, protein sources available so try to include them in your menus:

Meats such as lean beef, skinless chicken breast, white turkey, bison, venison, and pork tenderloin.

Fish such as salmon, tuna, cod, and mackerel.

Egg whites.

Low-fat dairy such as cottage cheese, Greek yogurt, Feta cheese, Parmesan cheese, or string cheese.

Non-animal sources such as tofu, tempeh, soy burgers, soy jerky, soy sausage, or seitan.

When you are on the go and don't have time to prepare a meal, you may want to even try a milk protein supplement such as whey, casein, or milk protein blends.

How much protein should you eat?

While not everyone likes to count calories and macronutrients, an easy method to figure your protein serving size would be to use the "eyeball" method. A serving size of protein for a woman is usually between 20 to 30 grams or the size of the palm of her hand. For men, a serving size would be 40 to 60 grams or two palms. Each serving of protein should be complimented with a serving of complex carbohydrates such as dark green leafy or colorful vegetables or metabolic boosting fruits. Metabolic boosting fruits may include apples, pears, grapefruits, or berries. Whole grains may compliment a couple of protein servings per day which may include oatmeal, brown or wild rice, or sweet potatoes.

Also include a serving of essential fats with your

protein: olive oil, flax seed, avocados, olives, walnuts, and almonds. The perfect diet plan combines all the healthy choices of protein, carbohydrates, and essential fats. Have a problem with fatigue? What about losing weight? Has it been difficult? Then eat lean protein meals throughout the day and see your energy skyrocket! More so, watch the scale go down and your clothes get baggy. Make sure you eat lean protein with all of your meals and discard the unbalanced diet. With balanced meals, you will be healthier, perform better, and even look better. Balanced meals are the perfect diet plan.

CHAPTER 15
LOW-FAT, HIGH-PROTEIN MEALS - 7 TIPS FOR A HEALTHIER BODY

We all know that in order to stay in shape we need to exercise regularly, get plenty of sleep, and eat right. One of the cornerstones of eating right is to avoid the evils of refined sugar, processed flour, and trans fats & saturated fats. But, what should you eat?

A great way to modify your diet in a way that keeps the pounds off is to eat more foods that are low in fat but high in protein. Once you know which foods to eat you can work them into each meal in unique and creative ways.

If you are looking for low-fat, high-protein meals, here are 7 tips for a healthier body:

1. What "low fat" means on labels:

Start your low-fat food journey by understanding how to read food label advertising properly. Marketers use a number of different terms to refer to low-fat content, but did you know that each one has a very specific meaning? Specifically:

* Reduced fat means the product has 25% less fat than the regular version of the same product

* Light means the product has 50% less fat than the regular version of the same product

* Low-fat means a product has less than 3 grams of fat per serving

2. Being "low fat" alone is not enough:

Remember, just because a food is low in fat (with less than 3 grams of fat per serving - see above), it may still be very high in sugar. Sugar can also add unwanted calories to your body, just as fat can.

3. Edamame:

Edamame is the Japanese word for immature soybeans prepared in the pod. They are a wonderful protein source, with 11g of protein for every half cup of beans. They also contain lots of other good-for-you stuff such as carbohydrates, omega fatty acids, manganese and vitamin K.

4. Low-fat cheese:

Everyone knows that cheese is delicious and is a great source of protein, but what about those fat calories? Some excellent low-fat cheeses are a great alternative to regular cheeses, including: part-skim mozzarella, string cheeses, farmers cheese, and Neufchatel.

5. High-protein, 100% whole grain bread:

Most white and some wheat breads are not very good for you. However, 100% whole great bread is a wonderful source of nutrition. For example, try Ezekiel 4:9 bread, which contains sprouted grain and no flour. Eat it with skinless chicken or turkey breast. Yummy!

6. Salmon:

Not only is salmon a wonderful, low-fat source of protein, but it contains the omega 3 fats which are so good for helping maintain the good type of cholesterol in your bloodstream.

7. Cottage cheese and plain yogurt:

Cottage cheese and plain yogurt are very good sources of protein, while having low fat content at the same time. But, do you find the taste a bit boring? If so, try them mixed with some dried fruits and chopped nuts to add some wonderful flavor.

CHAPTER 16
HOW IS THE QUALITY OF MID-DAY MEALS MAINTAINED

The Mid-day Meal Rules, 2015, notified by the Government of India (GoI) puts forth certain stipulations pertaining to the meals served to school children as a part of the Mid-day Meal Scheme. Among other things, it stresses on the nutritional standards and quality of mid-day meals; the latter being given due importance this time around.

Mid-day Meals Quality Guidelines

As far as the nutritional standards are concerned, it is stipulated that school lunch program should provide 450 calories and 12 g protein for primary students and 700 calories and 20 g protein for upper primary students. The implementing bodies, i.e., government schools, partnering non-profit organisations, etc., have to plan the menu accordingly. They can rotate the food items, or vegetables that are used in preparation of these food items, on a daily basis to ensure that the children get necessary nutrients in prescribed quantity.

Now, the personnel from an accredited lab can

evaluate hot cooked meal samples as and when deemed necessary to ensure its nutritional value and quality.

These new guidelines bring about a much-needed change to the ambitious scheme. The quality of food served to children deserves more attention, considering that the number of beneficiaries of this programme runs to the tune of over 100 million. Thus, not taking the quality aspect seriously will mean putting millions of children at risk and any untoward incident will affect the whole programme. The authorities need to ensure that such incidents do not occur; implementing stringent quality check regulations is one way to do this.

The notification makes it mandatory for every school to have a facility for storing raw materials and cooking meals without compromising on the hygiene. Additionally, it's important that the cooking staff maintains personal hygiene and wears gloves, masks, caps, etc., while cooking in order to avoid contamination. Also, there should be a proper arrangement of clean water and a waste disposal site in the vicinity.

The notification of new rules is a crucial step that will help in improving the quality of Mid-day Meal Programme. When a programme is being run at such a grand scale, it has to be constantly evaluated to minimize problems and make it more effective.

A lot goes into ensuring the quality of mid-day meals; right from careful selection of menu to proper hygiene.

Having said that, all these efforts are worth taking because the mid-day meal is at times, the only meal many of these children afford. In a country, where malnutrition is a chronic problem, the mid-day meal comes as a blessing in disguise.

CHAPTER 17
BALANCE YOUR LIFE - HAVING A BALANCED DIET

Understanding about a balanced diet growing up was simple. The meals pyramid was standard, and also you knew to eat a great deal of grains, some vegetables and fruits, a little bit of meat and dairy, and prevent the sugars and fats. Nonetheless, as science and medicine have evolved, the concept of your balanced diet has changed. Why does it matter? Why ought to you care? These are generally fair questions. This chapter will explain why a balanced diet is crucial, and methods for you to accomplish one.

First, you may need to understand that a balanced diet is incredibly crucial. One of the factors that everyone thinks of first when thinking about healthy diet is your bodyweight. If executed correctly, specifically with exercise, a balanced diet can allow you to maintain a balanced excess weight. If you will need to lose bodyweight, a balanced diet can support. On the other hand, the rewards of the balanced diet extend far beyond bodyweight. Eating the appropriate amounts of the perfect kinds of foods can also boost your energy. The correct blend of nutrition can provide you with vitamins and minerals that could cut down your chances of suffering from heart disease, diabetes and cancer. It has even been suggested that a healthy diet can increase your mood! All of these things are massive positive aspects to eating a healthy diet, no matter how obnoxious you may well discover the idea or execution.

How does one go about setting up a healthy diet? The first ting to appear at is the new and improved foods pyramid. The suggested servings have certainly changed, having a reduction in fruit and meats being suggested, along with an enhance in dairy. On the other hand, the meals pyramid is no longer static, either. If you're searching for some thing a little much more particular, firms like Excess weight Watchers and Jenny Craig might be quite helpful. It isn't just about fat loss with them. They also can allow you to set up a balanced diet to follow, and provide you with ideas on recipes and portions. Finally, you will need to usually talk to your doctor. They know you and your health greater than nearly anyone, and will be able to make suggestions that can enable you to be a lot more successful in achieving a wholesome diet.

Everyone would like to be a lot more nutritious. Fortunately, becoming a healthier individual is within reach should you make an effort to practice a healthy diet. Now that you know all the advantages of following a balanced diet, too as several methods to set one up, you no longer have any excuses.

CONCLUSION

It will perhaps astound you to learn that a person who is afflicted with the main causes of cancer (which constitute the real illness) would most likely die quickly unless he actually grew cancer cells. In this work, I provide evidence to this effect.

I further claim that cancer will only occur after all other defense or healing mechanisms in the body have failed. In extreme circumstances, exposure to large amounts of cancer-producing agents (carcinogens) can bring about a collapse of the body's defenses within several weeks or months and allow for rapid and aggressive growth of a cancerous tumor. Usually, though, it takes many years, or even decades, for these so-called "malignant" tumors to form.

Unfortunately, basic misconceptions or complete lack of knowledge about the reasons behind tumor growth have turned "malignant" tumors into vicious monsters that have no other purpose but to kill us in retaliation for our sins or abusing the body. However, as you are about to find out, cancer is on our side, not against us. Unless we change our perception of what cancer really is, it will continue to resist treatment, particularly the most "advanced" methods. If you have cancer, and cancer is indeed part of the body's complex survival responses and not a disease, as I suggest it is, you must find answers to the following pressing questions:

* What reasons coerce your body into developing cancer cells?

* Once you have identified these reasons, will you be able to change them? What determines the type and severity of cancer with which you are afflicted?

* If cancer is a survival mechanism, what needs to be done to prevent the body from taking recourse to such drastic defense measures?

* Since the body's original genetic design always favors the preservation of life and protection against adversities of any kind, why would the body permit self-destruction?

* Why do almost all cancers disappear by themselves, without medical intervention?

* Do radiation, chemotherapy and surgery actually cure cancer, or do cancer survivors heal due to other reasons, despite these radical, side-effect-loaded treatments?

* What roles do fear, frustration, low self-worth and repressed anger play in the origination and outcome of cancer?

* What is the spiritual growth lesson behind cancer?

To deal with the root causes of cancer, you must find satisfying and practical answers to the above questions. If you feel the inner urge to make sense of this life-changing event, (cancer that is), you most likely will recover from it. Cancer can be your greatest opportunity to help restore balance to all aspects of your life, but it can also be the harbinger of severe trauma and suffering. Either way you are always in control of your body.

To live in a human body, you must have access to a certain amount of life-sustaining energy. You may either use this inherent energy in a nourishing and self-sustaining or in a destructive and debilitating way. In case you consciously or unconsciously choose negligence or self-abuse over loving attention and self-respect, your body will likely end up having to fight for its life.

Cancer is but one of the many ways the body tries to change the way you see and treat yourself, including your body. This inevitably brings up the subject of spiritual health, which plays at least as important a role in cancer as physical and emotional reasons do.

Cancer appears to be a highly confusing and unpredictable disorder. It seems to strike the very happy and the very sad, the rich and the poor, the smokers and the non-smokers, the very healthy and the not so healthy. People from all backgrounds and occupations can have cancer. However, if you dare look behind the mask of its physical symptoms, such as the type, appearance and behavior of cancer cells, you will find that cancer is not as coincidental or unpredictable as it seems to be.

What makes 50% of the American population so prone to developing cancer, when the other half has no risk at all? Blaming the genes for that is but an excuse to cover up ignorance of the real causes. Besides, any good genetic researcher would tell you that such a belief is void of any logic and outright unscientific (as explained in the book).

Cancer has always been an extremely rare illness, except in industrialized nations during the past 40-50 years. Human genes have not significantly changed for thousands of years. Why would they change so drastically now, and suddenly decide to kill scores of people? The answer to this question is amazingly simple: Damaged or faulty genes do not kill anyone. Cancer does not kill a person afflicted with it! What kills a cancer patient is not the tumor, but the numerous reasons behind cell mutation and tumor growth. These root causes should be the focus of every cancer treatment, yet most oncologists typically ignore them. Constant conflicts, guilt and shame, for example, can easily paralyze the body's most basic functions, and lead to the growth of a cancerous tumor.

After having seen thousands of cancer patients over a period of three decades, I began to recognize a certain pattern of thinking, believing and feeling that was common to most of them. To be more specific, I have yet to meet a cancer patient who does not feel burdened by some poor self-image, unresolved conflict and worries, or past emotional trauma that still lingers in his/her subconscious. Cancer, the physical disease, cannot occur unless there is a strong undercurrent of emotional uneasiness and deep-seated frustration.

Cancer patients typically suffer from lack of self-respect or worthiness, and often have what I call an "unfinished business" in their life. Cancer can actually be a way of revealing the source of such inner conflict. Furthermore, cancer can help them come to terms with such a conflict, and even heal it altogether. The way to take out weeds is to pull them out along with their roots. This is how we must treat cancer; otherwise, it may recur eventually.

The following statement is very important in the consideration of cancer: "Cancer does not cause a person to be sick; it is the sickness of the person that causes the cancer." To treat cancer successfully requires the patient to become whole again on all levels of his body, mind and spirit. Once the cancer causes have been properly identified, it will become apparent what needs to be done to achieve complete recovery.

It is a medical fact that every person has cancer cells in the body all the time. These cancer cells remain undetectable through standard tests until they have multiplied to several billion. When doctors announce to their cancer patients that the treatments they prescribed had successfully eliminated all cancer cells, they merely refer to tests that are able to identify the detectable number of cancerous cells. Standard cancer treatments may lower the number of cancer cells to an undetectable level, but this certainly cannot eradicate all cancer cells. As long as the causes of tumor growth remain intact, cancer may redevelop at any time and at any rate.

Curing cancer has little to do with getting rid of a group of detectable cancer cells. Treatments like chemotherapy and radiation are certainly capable of poisoning or burning many cancer cells, but they also destroy healthy cells in the bone marrow, gastrointestinal tract, liver, kidneys, heart, lungs, etc., which often leads to permanent irreparable damage of entire organs and systems in the body. A real cure of cancer does not occur at the expense of destroying other vital parts of the body.

Each year, hundreds of thousands of people who were once "successfully" treated for cancer die from infections, heart attacks, liver failure, kidney failure and other illnesses because the cancer treatments generate a massive amount of inflammation and destruction in the organs and systems of the body. Of course, these causes of death are not being attributed to cancer. This statistical omission makes it appear we are making progress in the war against cancer. However, many more people are dying from the treatment of cancer than from cancer. A real cure or cancer is achievable only when the causes of excessive growth of cancer cells have been removed or stopped.

Power in the Word

Cancer is the second leading "cause" of death for Americans. According to the American Cancer Society, about 1.2 million cases will be diagnosed with cancer in the U.S. in 2008. More than 552,000 Americans will die of it. Among men, the top three cancer diagnoses are expected to be prostate cancer (180,400 cases), lung cancer (89,500 cases), and colorectal cancer (63,600). The leading types of cancer among women are breast cancer (182,800 cases), lung cancer (74,600), and colorectal cancer (66,600 cases).

Cancer is not just a word, but also a statement that refers to abnormal or unusual behavior of cells in the body. However, in quite a different context, cancer is referred to as a star sign. When someone tells you that you are a "cancer", are you going to tremble with fear of dying? It is unlikely, because your interpretation of being of the cancer sign does not imply that you have cancer, the illness. But if your doctor called you into his office and told you that you had cancer, you would most likely feel paralyzed, numb, terrified, hopeless, or all of the above.

The word "cancer" has the potential to play a very disturbing and precarious role, one that is capable of delivering a death sentence. Being a cancer patient seems to start with the diagnosis of cancer, although its causes may have been there for many years prior to feeling ill. Within a brief moment, the word "cancer" can turn someone's entire world upside down.

Who or what in this world has bestowed this simple word or statement with such great power that it can preside over life and death? Or does it really? Could it actually be that our collective, social belief that cancer is a killer disease, in addition to the aggressive treatments that follow diagnosis, are largely responsible for the current dramatic escalation of cancer in the Western hemisphere? Too far fetched, you might say! In this book, however, I will make the point that cancer can have no power or control over us, unless we unconsciously allow it to grow in response to the beliefs, perceptions, attitudes, thoughts, feelings we have, and the life choices we make.

Would we be just as afraid of cancer if we knew what caused it or at least understood what its underlying purpose is? Unlikely so! If truth were told, we would most probably do everything to remove the causes and, thereby, set the preconditions for the body to heal itself.

A little knowledge (which is what we call ignorance) is, in fact, a dangerous thing. Almost everyone, at least in the industrialized world, knows that drinking water from a filthy pond or polluted lake can cause life-threatening diarrhea, but still only few realize that holding on to resentment, anger and fear, or eating fast foods, chemical additives, and artificial sweeteners, is no less dangerous than drinking polluted water; it may just take a little longer to kill a person than tiny amoeba can.

Mistaken Judgment

We all know that if the foundation of a house is strong, the house can easily withstand external challenges, such as a violent storm. As we will see, cancer is merely an indication that there is something missing in our body and in life as a whole. Cancer shows that life as a whole (physical, mental and spiritual) stands on shaky grounds and is quite fragile, to say the least. It would be foolish for a gardener to water the withering leaves of a tree when he knows so well that the real problem is not where it appears to be, namely, on the symptomatic level (of withered leaves). By watering the roots of the plant, he naturally attends to the causative level, and consequently, the plant regenerates itself swiftly and automatically.

To the trained eye of a gardener, the symptom of withering leaves is not a dreadful disease. He recognizes that the dehydrated state of these leaves is but a direct consequence of withdrawn nourishment that they need in order to sustain themselves and the rest of the plant.

Although this example from nature may appear to be a simplistic analogy, it offers a profound understanding of very complex disease processes in the human body. It accurately describes one of the most powerful and fundamental principles controlling all life forms on the planet. However skilled we may have become in manipulating the functions of our body through the tools of allopathic medicine, this basic, highly evolved principle of evolution cannot be suppressed or violated without paying the hefty price of side-effect-riddled suffering and pain - physically, emotionally and spiritually.

I fervently challenge the statement that cancer is a killer disease. Furthermore, I will demonstrate that cancer is not a disease at all. Many people who received a "terminal" cancer sentence actually defied the prognosis and experienced total remission.

The Need for Answers

There is no cancer that has not been survived by someone, regardless how far advanced it was. If even one person has succeeded in healing his cancer, there must be a mechanism for it, just as there is a mechanism for creating cancer. Every person on the planet has the capacity for both. If you have been diagnosed with cancer, you may not be able to change the diagnosis, but it is certainly in your power to alter the destructive consequences that it (the diagnosis) may have on you. The way you see the cancer and the steps you take following the diagnosis are some of the most powerful determinants of your future wellness, or the lack of it.

The indiscriminate reference to "cancer" as being a killer disease by professionals and lay people alike has turned cancer into a disorder with tragic consequences for the majority of today's cancer patients and their families. Cancer has become synonymous to extraordinary suffering, pain and death. This is true despite the fact that 90-95 percent of all cancers appear and disappear out of their own accord. There is not a day that passes without the body making millions of cancer cells. Some people, under severe temporary stress make more cancer cells than usual and form clusters of cancerous cells that disappear again once they feel better. Secretions of the DNA's anticancer drug, Interleukin II, drop under physical and mental duress and increase again when relaxed and joyful. Thus, most cancers vanish without any form of medical intervention and without causing any real harm.

Right at this moment, there are millions of people walking around with cancers in their body without having a clue that they have them. Likewise, there are millions of people who heal their cancers without even knowing it. Overall, there are many more spontaneous remissions of cancer than there are diagnosed and treated cancers.

The truth is, relatively few cancers actually become "terminal." However, once diagnosed, the vast majority of all cancers are never even given a chance to disappear on their own. They are promptly targeted with an arsenal of deadly weapons of cell destruction such as chemotherapy drugs, radiation and the surgical knife. The problem with cancer patients is that, terrified by the diagnosis, they submit their bodies to all these cut/burn/poison procedures that, more likely than not, lead them to the day of final sentencing, "We have to tell you with our deepest regret there is nothing more that can be done to help you."

The most pressing question is not how advanced or dangerous a cancer is, but what we need to do to not end up dying from it. Why do some people go through cancer as if it were the flu? Are they just lucky or is there a mechanism at work that triggers the healing? In other words, what is that element that prevents the body from healing cancer naturally, or what is that hidden element that makes cancer so dangerous, if it is dangerous at all?

The answers to all these queries lie with the response of the person who has the cancer, and not with the degree of "viciousness" or advanced stage it appears to have progressed to. Do you believe that cancer is a disease? You will most likely answer with a "yes," given the 'informed' opinion that the medical industry and mass media have fed to the masses for many decades. Yet, the most pressing yet rarely asked question remains: "Why do you think cancer is a disease?" You may say: "Because I know cancer kills people every day." I would question you further: "How do you know that it is the cancer that kills people?" You would probably argue that most people who have cancer die, so obviously it must be the cancer that kills them. Besides, you may reason, all the expert doctors tell us so.

Let me raise another question, a rather strange one: "How do you know for sure that you are the daughter/son of your father and not of another man?" Is it because your mother told you so? What makes you think that your mother told you the truth? Probably because you believe her; and you have no reason not to. After all, she is your mother, and mothers do not lie about these things. Or do they? Although you will never really know that the person you believe to be your father is, in fact, your father, you nevertheless have turned what you subjectively believe into something that you just "know," into an irrefutable truth.

Although there is no scientific proof whatsoever that cancer is a disease (versus a survival mechanism), most people will insist that it is a disease because this is what they were told to believe. Yet their belief is only hearsay information based on other people's opinions. These other people heard it from someone else. Eventually, the "truth" of cancer being a disease can be traced to some doctors who expressed their subjective feelings or beliefs about what they observed and wrote about in some review magazines or medical reports. Other doctors agreed with their opinion, and before long, it became a "well-established" fact that cancer is a vicious illness that somehow gets hold of people in order to kill them. However, the truth of the matter may be quite different.

Wisdom of Cancer Cells

Cancer cells are not part of a malicious disease process. When cancer cells spread (metastasize) throughout the body, it is not their purpose or goal to disrupt the body's vitals functions, infect healthy cells and obliterate their host (the body). Self-destruction is not the theme of any cell unless, of course, it is old and worn-out and ready to be turned-over and replaced. Cancer cells, like all other cells, know that if the body dies, they will die as well. Just because some people assume that cancer cells are there to destroy the body does not mean cancer cells have such a purpose or ability.

A cancerous tumor is neither the cause of progressive destruction nor does it actually lead to the death of the body. There is nothing in a cancer cell that has even remotely the ability to kill anything. What eventually leads to the demise of an organ or the entire body is the wasting away of cell tissue resulting from continued deprivation of nutrients and life force. The drastic reduction or shutdown of vital nutrient supplies to the cells of an organ is not primarily a consequence of a cancerous tumor, but actually its biggest cause.

By definition, a cancer cell is a normal, healthy cell that has undergone genetic mutation to the point that it can live in an anaerobic surrounding (an environment where oxygen is not available). In other words, if you deprive a group of cells of vital oxygen (their primary source of energy), some of them will die, but others will manage to alter their genetic software program and mutate in a most ingenious way: the cells will be able to live without oxygen and derive some of their energy needs from such things as cellular metabolic waste products.

It may be easier to understand the cancer cells phenomenon when comparing it with the behavior of common microorganisms. Bacteria, for example, are divided into two main groups, aerobic and anaerobic, meaning, those that need to use oxygen and those that can live without it. This is important to understand since we have more bacteria in our body than we have cells. Aerobic bacteria thrive in an oxygenated environment. They are responsible for helping us with the digestion of food and manufacturing of important nutrients, such as B-vitamins. Anaerobic bacteria, on the other hand, can appear and thrive in an environment where oxygen does not reach. They break down waste materials, toxic deposits and dead, worn-out cells.

The body sees the cancer as being such an important defense mechanism that it even causes the growth of new blood vessels to guarantee the much-needed supply of glucose and, therefore, survival and spreading of the cancer cells. It knows that cancer cells do not cause but, prevent death; at least for a while, until the wasting away of an organ leads to the demise of the entire organism. If the trigger mechanisms for cancer (causal factors) are properly taken care of, such an outcome can be avoided.

It is commonly believed that our immune system protects us against cancer. However, this is only partially true. On the one hand, the immune system readily destroys the millions of cancer cells that a healthy human body produces as part of the daily turnover of 30 billion cells. On the other hand, the immune system takes no action to eradicate cancer cells that develop in response to a build up of toxins, congestion and emotional stress.

Cancers and all other tissues in the body are larded with cancer-killing white cells, such as T-cells. In the case of kidney cancer and melanomas, for example, white cells make up 50 per cent of the mass of the cancers. Since these T-cells easily recognize foreign or mutated cell tissue such as cancer cells, you would expect these immune cells to attack cancer cells right away. However, the immune system allows cancer cells to recruit it to actually increase and spread the cancer to other parts of the body. Cancer cells produce specific proteins that tell the immune cells to leave them alone and help them to grow

Why would the immune system want to collaborate with cancer cells to make more or larger tumors? Because cancer is a survival mechanism, not a disease. The body uses the cancer to keep deadly carcinogenic substances and caustic metabolic waste matter away from the lymph and blood and, therefore, from the heart, brain and other vital organs. Killing off cancer cells would in fact jeopardize its survival. Cleansing the body of accumulated toxins and waste products through the various cleansing methods advocated in my book Timeless Secrets of Health & Rejuvenation removes the need for cancer.

Cancer is not a disease; it is the final and most desperate survival mechanism the body has at its disposal. It only takes control of the body when all other measures of self-preservation have failed. To truly heal cancer and what it represents in a person's life we must come to the understanding that the reason the body allows some of its cells to grow in abnormal ways is in its best interest and not an indication that it is about to destroy itself. Cancer is a healing attempt by the body, for the body. Blocking this healing attempt can destroy the body. Supporting the body in its healing efforts can save it.

Do not go yet; One last thing to do

If you enjoyed this book or found it useful I'd be very grateful if you'd post a short review on it. Your support really does make a difference and I read all the reviews personally so I can get your feedback and make this book even better.

Thanks again for your support!

www.ingramcontent.com/pod-product-compliance
Lightning Source LLC
Chambersburg PA
CBHW060841220526
45466CB00003B/1187